PREDICTIVE SCIENCE

Healing the Future of Healthcare

Lalin L Laudis

notionpress
.com
INDIA · SINGAPORE · MALAYSIA

ISBN
Paperback 979-8-90479-255-8
Hardcase 979-8-90540-299-9

Dedicated

to

Vedhaa & Veena

This work is supported by

Visvesvaraya Post Doctoral Fellowship

Ministry of Electronics and Information Technology, MeiTY,

Govt. of India

Special Thanks to

St.Xavier's Catholic College of Engineering

Chunkankadai, Nagercoil.

Tamilnadu, India

Contents

SECTION I

The Dawn of Predictive Science

SECTION II

Biomarkers: The Language of Disease

SECTION V

Humanity, Ethics & Policy

SECTION VI

Beyond The Present: The Future of Human Health

Foreword

Rev. Fr. S. Godwin Selva Justus
Correspondent
St. Xavier's Catholic College of Engineering
Chunkankadai, Nagercoil – 629003

It gives me immense satisfaction and renewed enthusiasm to commend the author, Dr. Lalin L. Laudis, for his remarkable intellectual contribution to society through his scientific exploration in the field of healthcare. His book, *Predictive Science in Health Care*, is poised to become a valuable asset to humanity. The work thoughtfully traces the journey from traditional self-diagnostic methods, such as interpreting the heartbeat, to the advancements of artificial intelligence in modern medicine. While acknowledging the significant transformations in healthcare, the author insightfully highlights how treatments focused solely on symptoms can sometimes lead to unintended consequences in the body. In contrast, this book emphasizes the importance of preventing illness before it manifests.

With great prudence, the author successfully bridges ancient medical wisdom with contemporary technological innovations. He persuasively conveys that the human body continuously communicates through signals, and by learning to interpret these signals, one can prevent diseases before they develop into more serious conditions.

One of the most striking aspects of this work is its interdisciplinary richness. It seamlessly integrates insights from medicine, engineering, data science, and philosophy, offering a holistic perspective on healthcare. At the same time, the author remains deeply mindful of ethical and societal considerations, consistently upholding human dignity and social responsibility as central values.

Through this book, the author delivers a hopeful message: that advancements in technology have the potential to enhance both the longevity and quality of human life—not as a privilege for a few, but as a possibility accessible to all.

This work serves as an open invitation to individuals across disciplines to engage actively in the transformation of healthcare, with a focus on disease prevention. It stands as a source of inspiration for researchers, clinicians, engineers, policymakers, and students who aspire to reshape the future of human health. Moreover, it encourages readers to transcend conventional boundaries in envisioning and building a more effective healthcare system.

In endorsing this outstanding contribution, I wholeheartedly congratulate the author for his innovation, sense of social responsibility, unwavering commitment, and intellectual rigor.

Foreword

Very Rev. Fr. Satheesh Kumar
Correspondent
Mar Ephraem College of Engineering and Technology
Marthandam, Tamil Nadu, India

It is with immense joy, admiration, and intellectual appreciation that I write this foreword for *Predictive Science: Healing the Future of Healthcare* authored by Dr. Lalin L. Laudis. This remarkable work stands as a profound scholarly contribution to the emerging world of predictive healthcare, where medicine is no longer confined to treating disease after suffering begins, but evolves toward anticipating illness before it manifests. In many ways, this book represents not only a scientific study, but also a visionary philosophical reflection on the future of human health.

Dr. Lalin L. Laudis is a distinguished researcher who has been actively working in the field of Predictive Science for nearly a decade. His sustained research experience, intellectual dedication, and interdisciplinary engagement have given him deep insights into the transformation currently unfolding in healthcare systems worldwide. Over the years, he has explored predictive analytics, artificial intelligence, speech biomarkers, non-invasive diagnostics, digital health intelligence, and computational healthcare systems with remarkable academic commitment. This long engagement with predictive science is clearly reflected throughout the book, where every chapter carries the depth of experience, clarity of thought, and maturity of a seasoned researcher.

One of the most impressive dimensions of this work is the author's ability to bridge ancient medical wisdom with contemporary technological advancement. The book thoughtfully connects traditional pulse-based diagnostic understanding with modern artificial intelligence, machine learning, biosensing technologies, and digital twin systems. This synthesis demonstrates an intellectually courageous approach rarely found in contemporary scientific writing. The author recognizes that while technology has advanced tremendously, the fundamental principles of understanding the human body through signals, rhythms, and patterns have existed for centuries. Modern predictive science, as he convincingly explains, is not merely a technological revolution but also a rediscovery of timeless medical insight.

The intellectual framework of this book is exceptionally rich and interdisciplinary. Dr. Lalin does not approach healthcare as an isolated medical domain. Instead, he presents it as a convergence of medicine, engineering, artificial intelligence, computational modeling, signal processing, ethics, and philosophy. Such integrative thinking is essential in the present century, where scientific progress increasingly depends on collaboration across disciplines. Through this work, the author demonstrates how predictive healthcare can emerge only when diverse areas of knowledge work together in harmony.

The chapters discussing biomarkers, intelligent signal systems, speech analysis, pulse diagnostics, digital twins, machine learning, wearable biosensors, and predictive algorithms reveal not only technical expertise but also deep conceptual understanding. The author explains highly complex scientific concepts with clarity and intellectual elegance, making the book accessible to researchers, clinicians, engineers, policymakers, and students alike. His discussion on the body as an intelligent signal system is particularly insightful, emphasizing that disease does not begin suddenly but evolves gradually through detectable physiological deviations. Such perspectives redefine the philosophy of diagnosis itself.

Another remarkable aspect of this work is its emphasis on prevention as the highest form of medicine. Modern healthcare systems across the world remain largely reactive, responding to disease only after irreversible damage has occurred. Dr. Lalin challenges this paradigm with compelling scientific reasoning. He argues that predictive science enables humanity to shift from reaction to anticipation, from crisis management to intelligent prevention. This transition has enormous implications not only for medicine but also for economics, public health policy, and human well-being.

Equally commendable is the ethical awareness that runs throughout the book. The author does not glorify technology uncritically. Instead, he consistently emphasizes human dignity, privacy, responsibility, transparency, and equitable healthcare access. In an age where artificial intelligence is rapidly entering every aspect of human life, such ethical grounding is deeply important. The author reminds us that technology must remain a servant of humanity rather than its controller. This balance between scientific innovation and ethical responsibility gives the work exceptional academic value.

What makes this book especially inspiring is its visionary outlook. Dr. Lalin invites readers to imagine a future where healthcare becomes continuous, intelligent, personalized, and compassionate. A future where subtle biological signals can reveal disease risk years before symptoms appear. A future where predictive intelligence reduces suffering, improves quality of life, and extends healthy longevity. Such a vision reflects not only scientific imagination but also a profound concern for humanity.

The depth of research evident in this work deserves special appreciation. The author's decade-long involvement in predictive science has enabled him to develop insights that go beyond theoretical understanding. His reflections emerge from sustained engagement with real scientific challenges, emerging technologies, and interdisciplinary exploration.

This practical intellectual experience gives authenticity and strength to the arguments presented throughout the book.

I firmly believe that *Predictive Science: Healing the Future of Healthcare* will become an important academic and intellectual contribution in the years ahead. It has the potential to inspire future researchers, stimulate interdisciplinary innovation, and encourage society to rethink the very meaning of healthcare. This work will serve as a valuable guide for all those who aspire to participate in building a preventive, intelligent, and humane healthcare system for the future.

I wholeheartedly congratulate Dr. Lalin L. Laudis for this outstanding achievement. His scholarly rigor, originality of thought, scientific vision, and dedication to human welfare deserve the highest appreciation. May this book inspire deeper inquiry, meaningful innovation, and transformative progress in the field of predictive healthcare.

Preface

Humanity has always dreamed of defeating disease. From ancient healers reading pulses under candlelight to modern surgeons operating with robotic precision, we have travelled centuries powered by hope, courage, and curiosity. Yet, despite extraordinary advancements, a single truth has remained unchanged: **we wait for disease to arrive before fighting it**.

We have lived in a world where healthcare begins after suffering begins— where medicine responds to damage rather than preventing it, where diagnosis follows decline rather than predicting it.

But today, we stand on the threshold of a transformation that will redefine the meaning of health itself.

For the first time in human history, we possess the intelligence, the computing power, and the biological understanding required to **predict disease long before it manifests**. The body is no longer an enigma waiting to be interpreted through visible symptoms. Instead, it is a symphony of signals—electrical, acoustic, molecular, neural and emotional—that speak continuously, waiting to be heard.

Predictive Science is the field that listens to these hidden signals and translates them into foresight. It is the science that sees the unseen, hears the unheard, and acts before damage unfolds. It is the bridge between life as it is and life as it could be—longer, healthier, more dignified, and more humane.

This book is written not just as a scientific exploration, but as a vision of a future where:

- *healthcare becomes proactive rather than reactive,*
- *technology becomes compassionate rather than mechanical,*
- *disease becomes preventable rather than inevitable.*

A future where **every human being is protected by intelligence before pain demands attention**.

This work is my humble contribution to that vision—drawn from years of research in predictive analytics, speech biomarkers, non-invasive diagnosis, synthetic data modelling, nature-inspired optimization, and AI-driven medical intelligence.

May this book serve as a seed— a spark that ignites researchers, physicians, engineers, leaders, policymakers, and students to build a world where prediction is the greatest medicine and **Health becomes a Human Right, not a Human Fight.**

– Lalin L Laudis

How to Read This Book

This book is not meant to be read in haste. It is designed as a journey—one that moves across time, disciplines, and perspectives, connecting ancient wisdom with modern science and extending into the future of human health. While it follows a logical structure, it also invites reflection, pause, and personal interpretation. Readers are encouraged to approach it not merely as a source of information, but as a framework for rethinking healthcare itself.

The chapters progress from foundational philosophy to scientific depth, from historical insight to advanced technological vision. Early sections establish the shift from reactive medicine to predictive healing, grounding the reader in why such a transformation is necessary. These chapters may be read slowly, allowing the ideas to settle, as they form the conceptual backbone of everything that follows. They are intended to recalibrate how we think about disease, diagnosis, and the role of intelligence in medicine.

As the book moves forward, the language of biomarkers, signals, algorithms, and artificial intelligence becomes more prominent. Readers with a medical, engineering, or data science background may find these sections immediately familiar, while others may find them intellectually demanding. The chapters are written to remain accessible without oversimplifying complexity. Mathematical ideas, computational models, and technological concepts are explained through narrative rather than formula-heavy exposition, ensuring that understanding emerges gradually and intuitively.

The disease-specific chapters are structured to be both sequential and independent. A reader interested in a particular condition—such as Parkinson's disease, cardiovascular disorders, diabetes, or mental health—may choose to read those chapters independently without losing coherence. At the same time, reading them in sequence reveals a deeper pattern: that seemingly unrelated diseases often share predictive signatures, signal behaviors, and algorithmic principles. This realization is central to the philosophy of predictive science.

The later sections of the book shift focus from individual disease prediction to systems, ethics, policy, and the future of humanity. These chapters are intentionally reflective. They explore not only what can be done, but what should be done. Readers are invited to think critically about privacy, responsibility, equity, and the societal impact of predictive healthcare. These chapters do not aim to provide final answers, but to frame the right questions for the decades ahead.

Throughout the book, quotes appear at intervals. These are not decorative. They are intended as moments of stillness—points where the reader may pause, reflect, and connect the scientific narrative with human experience. The reader is encouraged to linger with these lines, as they often express in a single sentence what entire chapters attempt to explain.

This book may be read by students, researchers, clinicians, engineers, policymakers, and curious minds alike. Each reader will take something different from it. Some may focus on the science, others on the philosophy, and others on the future vision. There is no single correct way to read this book. What matters is not speed, but engagement.

Above all, this book is an invitation—to listen more closely to the body, to think more deeply about health, and to imagine a future where disease is no longer an unexpected fate but a preventable possibility. Read it with curiosity, patience, and openness. The ideas within are not meant to end on the page; they are meant to continue in thought, research, and action.

SECTION I

The Dawn of Predictive Science

Chapter 1

The New Era of Healthcare

From Reactive Treatment to Predictive Healing

The history of medicine is inseparably bound to human suffering. For thousands of years, disease has shaped civilizations, shortened lives, and tested the limits of human endurance. From ancient healers who relied on observation and intuition to modern physicians armed with imaging machines and pharmaceuticals, healthcare has largely followed the same underlying philosophy: intervene only after illness reveals itself. Pain, fever, paralysis, breathlessness, or visible dysfunction became the signal for action. By the time treatment began, the body had already crossed the threshold from balance to breakdown.

Even in the present age, surrounded by advanced hospitals and sophisticated medical technologies, this reactive mindset continues to dominate. A person seeks care only after chest pain begins, not while the heart silently weakens. Neurodegenerative diseases are diagnosed years after irreversible neuronal loss has occurred. Metabolic disorders are confirmed after long periods of unnoticed imbalance. Cancer is often discovered when structural changes become visible, not when the first molecular disruptions arise. We celebrate medical success stories while quietly accepting that intervention came late.

This approach is not a failure of effort or intelligence. It is a limitation of timing. Medicine, as practiced for centuries, has been fighting disease after it has already established itself.

"The greatest limitation of traditional medicine is not lack of treatment, but lateness of action."

A Silent Revolution Begins

A profound transformation is now unfolding—quietly, steadily, and decisively. It is not announced by dramatic breakthroughs alone, but by a gradual shift in how we understand the human body. This transformation is the emergence of Predictive Science, a discipline that does not wait for disease to manifest, but seeks to identify its earliest footprints long before symptoms appear.

The human body is not silent, nor is it random. It is a continuous generator of signals—electrical, chemical, mechanical, acoustic, and behavioral. Every heartbeat carries information about vascular health. Every breath reflects respiratory and metabolic balance. Speech patterns encode neurological integrity. Gait reveals musculoskeletal and cognitive coordination. Hormonal rhythms reflect internal regulation. These signals fluctuate subtly over time, often years before disease reaches a clinical stage.

Predictive Science is founded on the understanding that disease does not begin suddenly. It evolves gradually, following identifiable trajectories. Long before pain emerges, the body deviates from its healthy patterns. These deviations, once invisible, are now measurable. Advances in biosensing technologies, artificial intelligence, machine learning, and computational modelling allow us to capture, analyze, and interpret these early signals with unprecedented precision.

Healthcare is no longer confined to episodic testing or hospital visits. It is becoming continuous, personalized, and anticipatory. Intelligence is moving closer to the individual—embedded in wearables, home environments, mobile devices, and digital platforms that monitor physiological and behavioral patterns silently and consistently. The future of medicine is no longer centered on buildings or equipment alone, but on understanding trajectories rather than events.

"The body whispers before it screams. Prediction begins with learning how to listen."

A Future Without Fear

To imagine predictive healthcare is to imagine a world where uncertainty no longer dominates human health. In such a world, early warning replaces emergency response. Subtle changes in heart rhythm alert an individual months before a cardiac event. Slight variations in voice characteristics reveal neurodegenerative risk years before physical symptoms appear. Continuous metabolic sensing identifies diabetic tendencies without invasive testing. Retinal micro-variations indicate neurological or vascular disease long before vision is affected. Emotional and cognitive shifts are recognized early, allowing mental health intervention before crisis.

This is not a speculative future. Many of these capabilities already exist in early forms. Artificial intelligence models are learning to recognize patterns that human perception cannot detect. Machine learning systems identify correlations across thousands of variables simultaneously. Digital twins—virtual representations of human physiology—are being developed to simulate disease progression and test interventions safely. Nature-inspired algorithms optimize predictions by mimicking biological intelligence itself. Together, these technologies are redefining what it means to diagnose, treat, and ultimately prevent disease.

In this emerging paradigm, the role of the physician evolves. The focus shifts from responding to illness to guiding wellness. Medical decisions become informed not only by present conditions, but by projected futures. Healthcare becomes a dialogue between human judgment and computational foresight, grounded in ethics, responsibility, and personalization.

"Prediction does not remove uncertainty; it replaces fear with preparedness."

A New Philosophy of Healing

The most significant transformation brought by Predictive Science is philosophical rather than technological. It challenges the long-held belief that disease is an unavoidable interruption of life. Instead, it reframes illness as a process that can often be anticipated, redirected, or prevented entirely. Hospitals become centers for complex care rather than first points of contact. Diagnosis becomes a navigational tool rather than a verdict. Health becomes a dynamic state maintained through awareness rather than an assumption taken for granted.

This shift empowers individuals to become active participants in their own health. The body is no longer a passive recipient of treatment, but a continuously communicating system. Predictive Science restores agency, allowing people to understand their internal signals and respond before damage occurs. It transforms healthcare from an act of rescue into an act of preservation.

The journey that follows in this book will explore how this transformation is possible. It will move through ancient practices of pulse diagnosis, modern biomarkers, artificial intelligence, optimization algorithms, ethical considerations, and future visions of intelligent healthcare systems. At its core, however, the message remains simple and profound.

"The best cure is the one that is never needed."

We are entering an era where intelligence becomes medicine, where foresight becomes protection, and where health is no longer defended by reaction, but by understanding. This is the new era of healthcare—not defined by disease, but by the ability to prevent it.

And the future of that era begins with prediction.

Chapter 2

The Science of Prediction

From Reaction to Prevention

Prediction has always been central to human survival. Long before modern science emerged, humanity learned to anticipate danger by observing patterns—dark clouds before a storm, animal behavior before an earthquake, seasonal shifts before famine. Survival depended not on reacting to catastrophe, but on recognizing its earliest signs. Medicine, however, took a different path. While other sciences embraced anticipation, healthcare largely remained bound to reaction.

The idea that disease could be predicted before symptoms appear was once considered speculative. Illness was treated as an event rather than a process, an interruption rather than a trajectory. Yet biology does not operate in sudden leaps. Every disease evolves gradually, shaped by countless small deviations that accumulate over time. Prediction, therefore, is not an intrusion into medicine; it is a return to biological truth.

Predictive Science arises from this understanding. It is not a single technology or algorithm, but a way of thinking—a scientific philosophy that views health as a continuously evolving state and disease as a detectable deviation from equilibrium.

'Nothing in biology happens suddenly. Only our awareness does."

Prediction as a Scientific Principle

At its core, prediction is the ability to infer future states from present and past information. In scientific terms, it is the mapping of observed variables into future outcomes through models, patterns, and probabilities. In healthcare, this means interpreting physiological, molecular, behavioral, and environmental data to estimate the likelihood of disease before it manifests clinically.

The human body operates as a dynamic system governed by feedback, adaptation, and regulation. Heart rhythms adjust to physical demand, hormones respond to stress, neural circuits adapt to learning, and immune responses recalibrate constantly. Disease begins when these regulatory mechanisms drift away from balance. Importantly, this drift is measurable long before symptoms appear.

Predictive Science formalizes this concept through computational models that learn normal patterns and identify subtle deviations. Time-series analysis of physiological signals, probabilistic modeling of disease progression, and machine learning techniques allow the estimation of future health states based on current trends. Rather than asking whether disease is present, predictive systems ask how likely it is to emerge and how fast it may progress if no intervention occurs.

This approach fundamentally alters the nature of diagnosis. Traditional diagnosis confirms disease after it crosses a defined threshold. Predictive diagnosis identifies risk while the system is still reversible. It transforms diagnosis from a declaration into a warning.

"Diagnosis tells us what has happened. Prediction tells us what can still be prevented."

From Signals to Foresight

Every predictive system begins with signals. These signals may originate from the heart, brain, voice, blood, movement, sleep, or behavior. Individually, they may appear insignificant. Collectively, they form patterns that reflect the internal state of the body with remarkable accuracy. The challenge is not the absence of data, but the ability to interpret it meaningfully.

Modern predictive healthcare relies on the integration of signal processing, statistics, artificial intelligence, and biological insight. Raw signals are first transformed into features—measurable characteristics such as variability, frequency, symmetry, entropy, and correlation. These features capture the essence of physiological behavior without requiring invasive observation. Over time, patterns emerge that differentiate healthy trajectories from pathological ones.

Machine learning models learn these distinctions by analyzing large datasets across populations and individuals. They do not rely on fixed rules, but on adaptive learning, allowing them to improve as more data becomes available. Importantly, predictive models operate in probabilities rather than certainties. This probabilistic nature reflects biological reality, where outcomes are influenced by genetics, environment, lifestyle, and chance.

Prediction, therefore, is not about declaring inevitability. It is about quantifying risk. A predicted disease is not a sentence, but an opportunity—an invitation to intervene early, adjust behavior, modify treatment, and alter trajectory.

The transition from signals to foresight marks the turning point where medicine becomes intelligent rather than reactive. It allows healthcare systems to act before crises occur, conserving resources while preserving life quality.

"Prediction does not claim certainty. It offers choice."

Prevention as the Ultimate Outcome

The ultimate purpose of prediction is prevention. When disease risk is identified early, intervention becomes simpler, less invasive, and more humane. Lifestyle modifications, early therapies, monitoring strategies, and personalized guidance can redirect health trajectories without the need for aggressive treatment. Prevention, in this context, is not the absence of care, but its highest form.

Predictive Science shifts healthcare from episodic intervention to continuous guidance. Instead of waiting for symptoms to appear, individuals are supported throughout their lives with insights into their own physiological patterns. Health becomes an ongoing conversation rather than a crisis-driven response.

This shift has profound implications beyond individual well-being. Healthcare systems become more sustainable. Resources are allocated more efficiently. Chronic disease burden decreases. Quality of life improves not by extending survival alone, but by preserving function, dignity, and autonomy.

Most importantly, Predictive Science restores trust between humans and their bodies. Fear is replaced by understanding. Uncertainty is replaced by awareness. Medicine becomes not a reaction to suffering, but a partnership with life itself.

"The highest achievement of medicine is not curing disease, but ensuring it never needs to be cured."

As we move forward, the chapters ahead will explore how ancient civilizations practiced early forms of prediction, how biomarkers serve as the language of the body, how artificial intelligence amplifies human insight, and how technology can be guided ethically toward a future where health is anticipated rather than defended.

The science of prediction is not the end of medicine.

It is its evolution.

Chapter 3

Ancient Foundations of Predictive Healing

When Medicine Listened Before It Measured

Long before machines learned to calculate risk, long before algorithms processed signals, and long before medicine acquired laboratories and scanners, humanity had already begun to practice prediction. Ancient civilizations did not possess artificial intelligence, but they possessed something equally powerful: deep observation, patient listening, and an intuitive understanding that disease does not arrive suddenly. It announces itself quietly, through subtle changes in rhythm, behavior, temperature, emotion, and pulse. Ancient medicine was not reactive by design. It was fundamentally predictive.

In these early systems of healing, the physician was not merely a responder to illness, but a guardian of balance. Health was understood as harmony, disease as disharmony, and treatment as the restoration of equilibrium. The body was seen as a living system governed by rhythms and cycles, intimately connected to nature, seasons, emotions, and consciousness. Prediction was not expressed in numbers, but in patterns. Not in probabilities, but in perception.

Modern medicine often views ancient practices as symbolic or philosophical, yet when examined closely, many of these traditions reveal remarkably sophisticated predictive frameworks. They recognized early deviations long before disease became visible. They understood progression, prognosis, and prevention in ways that modern science is only now rediscovering through data and computation.

"Ancient medicine did not ask what disease you had. It asked where balance was lost."

The Body as a Rhythmic Intelligence

Across ancient medical traditions, a shared belief emerges: the human body speaks continuously through rhythm. Whether described as pulse, breath, energy flow, or elemental balance, rhythm was central to diagnosis. Health was defined not by static measurements, but by dynamic patterns over time.

In Ayurveda, the body was understood through the interplay of doshas—Vata, Pitta, and Kapha—each representing physiological and psychological tendencies. Disease was not an isolated event but a gradual shift in these governing forces. Subtle changes in pulse, digestion, sleep, voice, skin texture, and emotional state signaled the early stages of imbalance. The goal of the physician was to detect these changes before pathology took hold.

Similarly, Traditional Chinese Medicine viewed health as the smooth flow of Qi through meridians. Disruptions in flow manifested as changes in pulse quality, tongue appearance, facial complexion, and responsiveness to stimuli. These changes were not random; they followed predictable trajectories. A skilled practitioner could anticipate future illness by recognizing stagnation or excess long before pain or dysfunction appeared.

In Siddha medicine, which developed in the Indian subcontinent, diagnosis was deeply rooted in the concept of humoral balance and elemental harmony. The Siddhars emphasized observation over intervention, understanding that early correction required minimal effort, while delayed treatment demanded aggressive measures. The body was seen as a predictive system, revealing its future through present deviations.

Ancient Greek medicine, influenced by Hippocrates, echoed similar principles. Health was the balance of humors; disease was their imbalance. Prognosis was considered as important as diagnosis. Physicians were trained to anticipate outcomes, not merely respond to symptoms. Hippocrates himself emphasized observing the patient's environment, habits, and progression over time, recognizing that disease followed patterns that could be foreseen.

What unites these traditions is not a shared theory, but a shared method: continuous observation of subtle signals and interpretation of patterns over time. This is the essence of predictive science.

"To foresee disease is greater than to cure it." — attributed to Hippocratic thought

Pulse Reading: The First Predictive Signal

Among all ancient diagnostic methods, pulse reading stands as the most remarkable and misunderstood. Known as *Nadi Pariksha* in Ayurveda, pulse diagnosis was not limited to counting beats per minute. It was a sophisticated analysis of rhythm, force, depth, temperature, symmetry, and variability. Each quality conveyed specific information about organ function, metabolic state, emotional balance, and disease trajectory.

An experienced practitioner could differentiate dozens of pulse patterns, each associated with particular physiological tendencies. The pulse was felt at multiple depths, each layer corresponding to different systems of the body. Changes in pulse character were interpreted not as current disease alone, but as indicators of future imbalance. The pulse was a timeline, not a snapshot.

In Traditional Chinese Medicine, pulse diagnosis was equally elaborate. Practitioners assessed pulses at multiple positions and depths on both wrists, interpreting qualities such as slipperiness, wiriness, strength, and irregularity. These qualities were mapped to organ systems and energy states. Importantly, pulse diagnosis was predictive. A weak or irregular pulse might indicate future organ dysfunction even in the absence of symptoms.

Modern science now recognizes that the pulse carries vast physiological information. Heart rate variability, arterial stiffness, waveform morphology, and micro-oscillations are powerful predictors of cardiovascular, neurological, and metabolic health. What ancient physicians sensed through trained touch, modern sensors measure through electronics. The principle, however, remains unchanged.

"The pulse does not lie. It tells the story before the symptoms speak."

The ancient practice of pulse reading was not mystical. It was empirical, experiential, and cumulative. Knowledge was refined across generations through observation and outcome correlation. While it lacked mathematical formalization, it embodied the same logic that underpins modern predictive models: observe patterns, track deviations, anticipate outcomes.

Prediction Without Instruments

One of the most profound aspects of ancient predictive healing is that it functioned without instruments. Diagnosis relied on the physician's senses—touch, sight, hearing, and intuition sharpened through years of disciplined practice. Facial expressions, skin tone, voice modulation, posture, gait, sleep patterns, and emotional state were all diagnostic inputs.

Speech, for instance, was recognized as a window into neurological and emotional health. Ancient texts describe changes in voice clarity, speed, tone, and articulation as indicators of internal imbalance. Today, speech signal analysis is emerging as a powerful biomarker for Parkinson's disease, depression, and cognitive decline. The ancient insight precedes modern validation by centuries.

Similarly, gait and posture were observed for signs of weakness, stiffness, or imbalance. These observations are now formalized through motion capture and biomechanical analysis. Sleep patterns, appetite changes, and emotional fluctuations were considered early warning signs rather than secondary symptoms.

Ancient medicine treated the human being as a whole, not as a collection of isolated organs. Prediction emerged naturally from this holistic perspective. Disease was understood as a systemic process unfolding gradually across multiple domains.

"When the whole is understood, the future becomes visible."

Why Ancient Predictive Wisdom Was Lost

Despite its depth, ancient predictive medicine gradually gave way to reactive models. The rise of modern science emphasized measurement, reductionism, and specialization. These advancements brought undeniable progress—surgical precision, pharmacological breakthroughs, and diagnostic imaging—but they also narrowed focus. Medicine became increasingly concerned with identifying disease entities rather than understanding disease trajectories.

The complexity of ancient systems, difficult to standardize and quantify, made them incompatible with industrialized healthcare models. As a result, prediction was replaced by confirmation, prevention by intervention. The intuitive intelligence of observation was overshadowed by the authority of tests.

Yet this shift came at a cost. Chronic diseases rose. Healthcare systems became overwhelmed. Prevention lagged behind treatment. Only now, as data science and artificial intelligence mature, is medicine regaining the tools needed to formalize what ancient healers intuitively knew.

The Return of Predictive Healing

Modern predictive science does not replace ancient wisdom; it completes it. Artificial intelligence provides the scale and precision that ancient practitioners lacked. Sensors capture what fingers once felt. Algorithms formalize what intuition once inferred. Data validates what experience once suggested.

In many ways, predictive science represents a return rather than a departure. It brings medicine back to its original purpose: to foresee, to prevent, and to preserve balance. The difference is that today, prediction can be shared, standardized, validated, and scaled across populations.

The ancient physician and the modern data scientist are not adversaries. They are partners separated by time. Both seek the same truth: that disease begins quietly, progresses predictably, and can be altered if recognized early.

"The future of medicine lies not in abandoning the past, but in understanding it deeply."

As this book moves forward, the next chapters will explore how these ancient insights are translated into biomarkers, algorithms, and intelligent systems. The pulse becomes a waveform, the voice becomes a signal, balance becomes a dataset, and intuition becomes a model. Yet the essence remains unchanged.

Prediction has always been the highest form of healing.

Only now do we have the tools to honor it fully.

Chapter 4

Pulse Reading: The First Predictive Diagnostic Tool

Listening to the Rhythm of Life

Among all the diagnostic tools humanity has ever developed, none is as ancient, intimate, and revealing as the pulse. Long before imaging devices illuminated organs and laboratories decoded blood chemistry, healers placed their fingers gently on the wrist and listened. In that quiet act lay an extraordinary truth: the pulse is not merely a beat—it is a narrative. It carries within it the story of the heart, the vessels, the organs, the mind, and the future.

Pulse reading is perhaps the earliest form of predictive medicine. It required no instruments, no electricity, no algorithms. Yet it enabled physicians to assess health, anticipate disease, and guide intervention with remarkable accuracy. Modern medicine often dismisses this practice as subjective, but contemporary science is now uncovering what ancient healers intuitively knew: the pulse is a high-dimensional physiological signal, rich with predictive information.

To understand pulse reading is to understand that the body never stops communicating. Every heartbeat reflects the state of circulation, neural regulation, hormonal balance, emotional stress, and metabolic demand. The pulse does not simply respond to disease; it evolves with it. It changes before symptoms appear, shifts before organs fail, and warns before collapse.

"The pulse is the voice of the heart,
and the heart is the witness of the future."

Ancient Pulse Wisdom Across Civilizations

In Ayurveda, pulse diagnosis—*Nadi Pariksha*—was regarded as a refined art and a rigorous science. Practitioners were trained for years to sense subtle differences in pulse quality using three fingers placed at specific positions on the wrist. Each finger corresponded to physiological principles governing the body. The pulse was assessed at different depths, revealing information about superficial and deep systems. Variations in rhythm, strength, smoothness, irregularity, temperature, and tension were interpreted as signs of imbalance.

Importantly, Ayurvedic pulse reading was not limited to identifying existing disease. It was explicitly predictive. A skilled practitioner could sense early disturbances in doshic balance long before illness manifested. These disturbances, if corrected early, required minimal intervention. If ignored, they progressed into structural disease.

Traditional Chinese Medicine developed an equally sophisticated pulse system. Practitioners evaluated pulses at multiple positions on both wrists, interpreting dozens of pulse qualities such as wiry, slippery, floating, deep, rapid, or slow. Each quality reflected the state of specific organs and energetic pathways. Pulse diagnosis was combined with observation of tongue, face, voice, and posture to construct a complete picture of health.

In Siddha medicine, pulse reading was deeply integrated with elemental theory. The pulse was understood as the outward expression of internal elemental balance. Variations were linked to organ systems, digestion, respiration, and mental state. The Siddhars emphasized prognosis, often predicting disease progression based on pulse characteristics even in asymptomatic individuals.

Ancient Greek physicians, though less formalized in pulse taxonomy, placed significant emphasis on pulse rhythm and strength. Hippocratic texts describe pulse observation as essential to prognosis. Galen later expanded this understanding, categorizing pulse variations and correlating them with disease states.

Across these traditions, a unifying principle emerges: the pulse is dynamic, contextual, and predictive. It is not a static measurement, but a living signal shaped by time.

"To read the pulse is to read the present as it becomes the future."

What the Pulse Truly Represents

From a modern physiological perspective, the pulse is a complex waveform generated by the interaction of cardiac contraction, arterial elasticity, neural control, blood viscosity, and peripheral resistance. Each heartbeat sends a pressure wave through the arterial system. The shape, timing, and variability of this wave carry extensive information about cardiovascular and systemic health.

Heart rate variability reflects autonomic nervous system balance. Arterial stiffness alters pulse wave velocity. Micro-irregularities reveal arrhythmias or early cardiac dysfunction. Changes in pulse amplitude reflect vascular health, hydration, and metabolic state. Emotional stress, inflammation, and endocrine imbalance all leave signatures in the pulse.

What ancient physicians sensed through touch, modern science measures through sensors. Pulse oximeters, photoplethysmography, arterial tonometry, and wearable biosensors now capture pulse signals continuously. Artificial intelligence models analyze waveform morphology, frequency components, and nonlinear dynamics to predict disease risk.

Yet the foundational insight remains unchanged: the pulse reflects the integrated state of the body. It is not limited to the heart alone.

It mirrors neurological regulation, emotional stress, respiratory efficiency, and systemic resilience.

The pulse, therefore, is not merely diagnostic. It is prognostic.

"The heart does not beat in isolation.
It beats in dialogue with the entire body."

Pulse as a Timeline, Not a Snapshot

One of the most profound differences between ancient pulse reading and modern vital sign measurement lies in perspective. Modern medicine often treats the pulse as a number—beats per minute—recorded at a single moment. Ancient medicine treated the pulse as a story unfolding over time.

Pulse characteristics were observed repeatedly across days, seasons, emotional states, and life stages. Patterns mattered more than absolute values. A gradually weakening pulse indicated future decline. Increasing irregularity signaled impending dysfunction. Subtle changes, though not alarming in isolation, became meaningful when tracked over time.

This temporal understanding aligns precisely with modern predictive modeling. Disease prediction relies on trend analysis rather than isolated readings. Continuous monitoring reveals trajectories that snapshots cannot. Wearable devices, combined with AI, are now recreating this ancient wisdom at scale.

Digital health systems track pulse signals continuously, learning individual baselines and detecting deviations unique to each person. Prediction becomes personalized rather than generalized. Intervention becomes timely rather than delayed.

The ancient physician relied on memory and intuition to track these changes. The modern system relies on data and algorithms. Both seek the same outcome: early awareness.

Why Pulse Reading Was Marginalized

Despite its depth, pulse reading gradually lost prominence in mainstream medicine. The reasons were not scientific failure, but structural transformation. Industrial medicine favored standardized, reproducible measurements. Pulse reading required training, experience, and interpretation. It resisted mechanization.

As laboratories and imaging advanced, medicine shifted toward visible pathology. The subtlety of early imbalance was overshadowed by the certainty of confirmed disease. Prognosis became secondary to diagnosis. Prediction yielded to verification.

Yet the cost of this shift became evident over time. Chronic diseases surged. Healthcare systems became reactive and expensive. Prevention lagged behind treatment. Only now, with the rise of computational power, is medicine able to return to prediction without sacrificing standardization.

The Pulse in the Age of Artificial Intelligence

Modern predictive science is rediscovering the pulse with new eyes. High-resolution pulse sensors capture waveforms far beyond human tactile perception. AI models analyze thousands of pulse features simultaneously. Patterns once felt intuitively are now mathematically represented.

Research shows that pulse-based features can predict cardiovascular disease, diabetes, sepsis, stress disorders, and even neurological conditions. Combined with speech, movement, and metabolic data, pulse signals become part of a multidimensional predictive framework.

In this convergence, ancient wisdom finds validation. The pulse once read by fingers is now read by algorithms. What was once experiential becomes empirical. What was once local becomes global.

"Technology did not replace ancient medicine. It gave it a voice loud enough for the world to hear."

A Bridge Between Past and Future

Pulse reading stands as a bridge between ancient healing and modern predictive science. It reminds us that the body has always been predictive. The limitation was never the signal, but our ability to interpret it.

As this book progresses, the pulse will reappear in new forms—heart rate variability, photoplethysmography, waveform analytics, wearable sensors, and AI-driven prediction models. Yet its essence remains unchanged.

The pulse is the rhythm of life.

It is the first signal we perceive at birth and the last to fade at death. Between these moments, it tells a story—if we learn how to listen.

Prediction did not begin with machines. It began with the pulse.

Chapter 5

The Human Body as an Intelligent Signal System

When Biology Becomes Information

The human body is often described as a machine, a structure of organs, tissues, and biochemical reactions working together to sustain life. Yet this description, while convenient, is profoundly incomplete. A machine functions through commands and components. The human body functions through signals. Every moment of life is orchestrated by an invisible conversation unfolding across electrical impulses, chemical gradients, mechanical vibrations, acoustic patterns, and rhythmic oscillations. To understand health and disease, one must first understand this language.

Long before disease manifests as pain or dysfunction, it expresses itself as a change in signals. The body does not fail suddenly; it drifts. It deviates quietly from its natural equilibrium, leaving traces in rhythms that most people never notice. Predictive Science is founded on a simple yet transformative realization: the body is not only biological—it is informational. It senses, processes, adapts, and communicates continuously. In doing so, it reveals its future long before it arrives.

"Life is not sustained by organs alone, but by the signals that bind them together."

Signals as the Foundation of Life

At the most fundamental level, life is a phenomenon of communication. Cells communicate with one another through chemical messengers. Neurons communicate through electrical impulses. Organs coordinate their function through feedback loops. The heart listens to the brain. The immune system listens to inflammation. Hormones listen to stress, sleep, and emotion. Nothing in the body operates in isolation. Every system responds to information it receives from other systems.

These signals exist across multiple domains. Electrical signals govern neural activity and muscle contraction. Mechanical signals reflect movement, posture, and circulation. Chemical signals regulate metabolism, immunity, and growth. Acoustic signals emerge through speech, breathing, and internal vibrations. Thermal signals reveal metabolic efficiency and inflammation. Behavioral signals reflect cognitive and emotional states. Together, these form a dense, multidimensional network of information.

Importantly, signals are not static. They fluctuate, adapt, and evolve in response to internal and external conditions. Health is characterized by flexibility and adaptability. Disease, in contrast, is marked by rigidity, loss of variability, and persistent deviation from normal patterns. This distinction is subtle but critical. A healthy heart does not beat like a metronome; it varies intelligently. A healthy nervous system does not respond uniformly; it adapts contextually. Variability is not noise—it is intelligence.

Ancient physicians sensed this truth intuitively. Modern science is now confirming it mathematically. Reduced variability in physiological signals is a hallmark of aging and disease. Heart rate variability declines before cardiovascular events. Neural signal complexity decreases before cognitive impairment. Gait variability changes before neurological disorders become clinically evident. These changes occur long before structural damage appears.

"Disease does not begin with failure. It begins with loss of adaptability."

The Body as a Distributed Intelligence

The intelligence of the human body is not centralized in the brain alone. It is distributed across networks that sense, respond, and learn continuously. The gut contains its own neural system. The immune system remembers past threats. Muscles adapt to repeated movement. Even cells exhibit decision-making behavior in response to their environment. This distributed intelligence allows the body to maintain balance in a constantly changing world.

Predictive Science views the body as a complex adaptive system. Such systems are defined not by linear cause-and-effect relationships, but by interactions, feedback loops, and emergent behavior. A small change in one part of the system can produce large effects elsewhere. Stress alters hormonal balance. Hormonal imbalance affects metabolism. Metabolic disruption influences cardiovascular health. Cardiovascular dysfunction impacts brain perfusion. The chain is continuous and interconnected.

Signals act as messengers across this network. They carry information about load, stress, damage, adaptation, and recovery. Importantly, the same signal may have different meanings depending on context. A rapid heartbeat during exercise is healthy adaptation. The same rhythm at rest may signal pathology. Prediction, therefore, requires contextual intelligence rather than isolated measurement.

Modern AI systems excel at this type of interpretation. They analyze relationships across signals, time, and conditions. They learn individual baselines and detect deviations unique to each person. This personalized interpretation mirrors the ancient physician's understanding that health cannot be defined by universal thresholds alone.

"The body does not follow averages. It follows its own logic."

From Signal Breakdown to Disease Emergence

Disease emerges when signal integrity is compromised. This breakdown may occur through persistent stress, genetic predisposition, environmental exposure, lifestyle imbalance, or aging. Initially, the body compensates. Feedback mechanisms adjust to maintain function. Over time, compensation becomes insufficient. Signals lose coordination. Variability decreases. Noise increases. Feedback loops destabilize. Only then do symptoms appear.

Consider neurodegenerative diseases. Long before neurons die, communication between neural networks becomes inefficient. Signal timing shifts. Speech patterns subtly change. Motor coordination becomes less fluid. These changes are detectable through signal analysis years before diagnosis. Similarly, cardiovascular disease begins with altered vascular signaling long before arteries are visibly blocked. Metabolic disorders begin with subtle insulin signaling dysfunction long before glucose levels cross diagnostic thresholds.

Traditional medicine often intervenes after structural damage is confirmed. Predictive Science intervenes when signal integrity begins to decline. This distinction defines the difference between prevention and repair.

The challenge lies not in collecting signals, but in interpreting them meaningfully. The human body produces enormous volumes of data. Without intelligence, data becomes noise. Predictive systems transform this noise into insight by identifying which signal changes matter, how they interact, and what they imply about future states.

This is where artificial intelligence becomes essential. AI does not replace biological understanding; it augments it. It allows us to see patterns across dimensions and timescales beyond human perception. It restores to medicine what industrialization took away: the ability to perceive early deviation.

"Signals are not symptoms. They are warnings."

The Return to Listening

The recognition of the body as an intelligent signal system represents a return to listening. Ancient medicine listened through touch and observation. Modern predictive science listens through sensors and algorithms. The method has changed, but the principle remains identical. Health reveals itself continuously. Disease announces itself quietly.

When medicine learns to listen again—deeply, continuously, and intelligently—it transforms. Diagnosis becomes anticipation. Treatment becomes guidance. Healthcare becomes preservation.

As this book moves forward, each chapter will explore specific signals in greater depth: pulse, speech, neural activity, biochemical markers, movement, and behavior. Each will be treated not as an isolated measurement, but as part of an integrated language spoken by the body.

Prediction begins not with machines, but with recognition. Recognition that the body is intelligent.

Recognition that signals carry meaning. Recognition that the future is already present—encoded quietly in the rhythms of life.

"The future of health is not hidden. It is simply unheard."

Chapter 6

Digital Twins in Medicine

Simulating Life Before It Changes

For centuries, medicine learned by observing life as it unfolded. Physicians watched symptoms appear, progress, and resolve—or fail to resolve. Every intervention carried uncertainty because it was applied to a living body without knowing exactly how that body would respond. Treatment was, in many ways, an informed gamble. Even today, despite extraordinary advancements, medicine often proceeds by trial and adjustment, learning outcomes only after decisions have already been made.

Digital twins represent a radical departure from this tradition. They introduce the possibility of learning before acting, of simulating health and disease in silico before intervening in vivo. A digital twin is not merely a computer model or a static representation of anatomy. It is a living computational counterpart of a human being, continuously updated with real-world data, capable of evolving, adapting, and predicting future states.

In this concept lies one of the most transformative ideas in the future of healthcare: the ability to test the future safely.

"The most humane medicine is the one that learns without causing harm."

From Mechanical Models to Living Mirrors

Early medical models were simplistic. Organs were represented as isolated components, equations approximated physiological behavior, and averages stood in for individuals. These models were useful, but limited. They could not capture the complexity, individuality, and adaptability of a living human system.

A digital twin changes this fundamentally. It mirrors not just structure, but behavior. It integrates signals from multiple domains—cardiovascular rhythms, neural activity, metabolic markers, genetic predispositions, environmental exposure, lifestyle patterns, and even emotional indicators. As real-world data flows into the system, the twin updates continuously, reflecting the evolving state of the person it represents.

This dynamic mirroring allows the twin to simulate what might happen next. How will the heart respond to sustained stress? How will glucose regulation change with altered sleep patterns? How will disease progress if intervention is delayed? How will a specific medication affect this individual rather than an average patient?

Digital twins shift medicine from population-based inference to individualized foresight. They transform uncertainty into scenario analysis.

What makes this possible is the convergence of predictive science disciplines: artificial intelligence to learn patterns, signal processing to extract meaningful features, computational physiology to model interactions, and high-performance computing to simulate time-dependent behavior. The twin becomes a bridge between data and decision.

"A digital twin is not a prediction of fate. It is a rehearsal of possibility."

Personalized Futures and Preventive Intelligence

The most profound impact of digital twins lies in prevention. When disease trajectories can be simulated early, intervention no longer depends on waiting. Subtle deviations detected in physiological signals can be projected forward, revealing future risk long before damage occurs. The twin allows clinicians and individuals to explore "what-if" scenarios safely. What if lifestyle remains unchanged? What if stress increases? What if early therapy is introduced now rather than later?

In cardiovascular care, digital twins can simulate arterial stiffness progression, arrhythmia risk, and heart failure development. In neurology, they can model cognitive decline trajectories based on speech, gait, and neural signals. In metabolic health, they can project diabetes risk based on behavior and biochemical trends. In oncology, digital twins may one day simulate tumor evolution and treatment response without exposing the patient to unnecessary harm.

This capability fundamentally alters decision-making. Treatment becomes proactive rather than reactive. Interventions become personalized rather than standardized. The role of the physician evolves from responder to guide, from crisis manager to architect of long-term wellness.

Importantly, digital twins do not replace human judgment. They augment it. They offer insight, not authority. The final decision remains human, informed by computational foresight rather than constrained by uncertainty.

"The future is no longer guessed. It is simulated."

The Ethics and Philosophy of Simulated Life

The idea of creating a digital counterpart of a human being raises profound ethical and philosophical questions. If a digital twin can predict disease, who owns that knowledge? If it reveals future risk, how should that information be communicated? Can prediction create anxiety as easily as it creates empowerment?

Predictive science must navigate these questions carefully. A digital twin must serve the individual, not control them. Transparency, consent, and interpretability are essential. The purpose of simulation is not surveillance, but support. Not control, but care.

There is also a deeper philosophical implication. Digital twins challenge the notion that the future is unknowable. They suggest that while fate may not be fixed, trajectories are detectable. This does not eliminate free will; it enhances it. When individuals understand their future risk, they gain the power to change it.

In this sense, digital twins restore agency. They return responsibility to the individual while providing guidance rooted in evidence rather than fear. They embody the highest ideal of predictive medicine: to inform without alarming, to guide without dictating.

"Knowledge of the future is meaningful only if it preserves freedom in the present."

A Glimpse Into the Future of Healthcare

In the coming decades, digital twins will likely become as fundamental to healthcare as medical records are today. Every individual may possess a continuously updated digital health companion, silently learning, simulating, and advising. Hospitals may consult twins before procedures. Physicians may test treatments virtually before prescribing them. Public health systems may simulate population-wide interventions safely before implementation.

The hospital of the future may not be a place of first response, but a center of complex intervention guided by predictive intelligence. Primary care may shift toward continuous digital companionship. Emergency medicine may become rarer as prevention becomes precise.

Digital twins will not eliminate disease. But they will reduce surprise. They will replace reaction with readiness. They will allow medicine to fulfill its highest promise—not merely to save life, but to protect it.

The human body has always been predictive.

Digital twins simply give it a mirror.

"The future of medicine lies not in reacting to reality, but in understanding it before it arrives."

As we move forward, the next chapter will explore how raw biological data becomes meaningful prediction—how signals transform into medicine, and how data itself becomes the new therapeutic medium.

Chapter 7

Data as the New Medicine

When Information Heals Before Intervention

For most of medical history, medicine arrived in tangible forms—herbs, compounds, pills, injections, surgeries. Healing was associated with substances and procedures, something that could be administered, ingested, or performed. Yet beneath every successful treatment lay an invisible factor more powerful than the drug itself: information. A correct diagnosis, a timely decision, an accurate understanding of the body's state—these determined outcomes as much as, if not more than, the intervention.

In the emerging era of predictive science, this invisible factor steps into the foreground. Data itself becomes medicine. Not metaphorically, but functionally. Information no longer merely supports treatment; it actively prevents disease, guides intervention, and reshapes the trajectory of health. When interpreted intelligently, data heals not by altering chemistry directly, but by altering decisions early enough to avoid damage altogether.

"The most powerful medicine is the one that changes the future before the body needs repair."

From Measurement to Meaning

The modern human body is surrounded by data. Heartbeats are logged by wearables. Sleep cycles are tracked by sensors embedded in mattresses and watches. Speech is recorded by devices that capture tone, rhythm, and hesitation. Movement is measured through accelerometers. Blood chemistry is digitized. Genetic sequences are stored as datasets. Medical histories, once scattered across paper files, now exist as structured records.

Yet raw data alone has no healing power. Numbers do not cure. Signals do not prevent. It is meaning—extracted, contextualized, and interpreted—that transforms data into medicine. Predictive science is built on this transformation. It is the discipline that converts data into foresight and foresight into action.

The distinction between traditional data use and predictive data use is profound. Conventional medicine often relies on threshold-based interpretation. A value crosses a predefined limit, and disease is declared. Predictive medicine, by contrast, focuses on trends, variability, correlations, and deviation from personal baselines. It asks not whether a number is abnormal, but whether its trajectory suggests future risk.

This shift mirrors a deeper truth about biology. Health is not a fixed point; it is a moving pattern. Disease does not appear suddenly; it emerges gradually. Data, when viewed longitudinally, reveals these patterns. It allows medicine to detect disease in its formative stages, when intervention is simplest and most effective.

"Health is not a number. It is a pattern unfolding over time."

Why Data Can Prevent Disease

One of the most striking realities of modern healthcare is that many chronic diseases are predictable long before diagnosis. Cardiovascular disease develops over decades. Neurodegenerative disorders progress silently for years. Metabolic syndromes evolve gradually. Mental health conditions often emerge from subtle behavioral and physiological shifts.

Data captures these shifts. Changes in heart rate variability precede cardiac events. Alterations in speech patterns signal neurological decline.

Variations in sleep and activity reflect metabolic imbalance. Emotional tone embedded in voice and behavior reveals psychological distress. These signals, individually modest, become powerful when integrated.

Artificial intelligence enables this integration. Machine learning models analyze thousands of data points simultaneously, identifying relationships no human clinician could track unaided. Importantly, these models learn continuously. As more data is collected, predictions improve. Medicine evolves in real time.

This capability transforms prevention from a generalized recommendation into a personalized strategy. Instead of advising everyone to follow the same guidelines, predictive systems tailor guidance to individual risk profiles. Intervention becomes specific, timely, and proportionate.

In this context, data functions as medicine by influencing behavior, guiding lifestyle, optimizing therapy, and preventing escalation. No chemical compound is administered, yet disease is avoided. No surgery is performed, yet function is preserved.

"Prevention is not the absence of treatment. It is treatment delivered early enough to be invisible."

Data-Driven Medicine and the End of Averages

Traditional medicine has relied heavily on population averages. Clinical trials establish what works for the majority. Guidelines recommend interventions based on generalized risk. While this approach has saved countless lives, it struggles with individuality. The human body does not conform neatly to averages. Genetics, environment, behavior, and psychology shape unique trajectories.

Data-driven medicine challenges this limitation. By continuously collecting individual data, predictive systems learn what is normal for a specific person. Deviations are detected relative to that baseline, not an abstract norm. This personalization is critical. A heart rate considered normal for one individual may signal distress in another. A sleep pattern benign for one may indicate pathology for someone else.

Digital twins amplify this personalization by simulating individual futures rather than population outcomes. Data feeds these twins, updating predictions dynamically. Medicine becomes adaptive rather than static.

This shift has profound implications. Misdiagnosis decreases. Overtreatment declines. Resources are allocated more efficiently. Patients feel seen not as cases, but as individuals.

"The future of medicine belongs not to the average patient, but to the individual story."

Data Ethics and the Responsibility of Prediction

As data assumes the role of medicine, ethical responsibility deepens. Predictive insight carries power. Knowing future risk can empower, but it can also burden. Data must be handled with care, transparency, and respect for autonomy.

Predictive medicine must avoid determinism. A prediction is not a verdict. It is a probability, shaped by variables that can often be altered. Communication becomes as important as computation. Individuals must understand not only what data suggests, but what choices remain available.

Privacy is equally critical. Health data is deeply personal. As data becomes medicine, protecting it becomes equivalent to protecting physical well-being. Secure systems, consent-driven sharing, and ethical governance are essential.

The goal of predictive data use is not surveillance, but support. Not control, but care. Data should serve as a guide, not a judge.

"Prediction without compassion is not medicine."

A Glimpse of the Future

In the decades ahead, data will increasingly replace invasive diagnostics. Continuous monitoring will reduce the need for episodic testing. Hospitals will rely on predictive dashboards rather than emergency alarms. Physicians will consult models that simulate outcomes before making decisions. Individuals will engage with personalized health companions that translate data into understandable guidance.

Public health systems will shift from reactive response to anticipatory planning. Disease outbreaks will be forecasted earlier. Resource allocation will become proactive. Healthcare costs will decline as prevention outpaces treatment.

Most importantly, the relationship between humans and medicine will change. Health will no longer be something checked occasionally, but something understood continuously. Data will become a quiet guardian, working in the background to preserve balance.

The pill, the scalpel, and the machine will remain essential. But they will be used less frequently, more precisely, and with greater wisdom. Data will guide when and how they are deployed.

"The medicine of the future will not be swallowed. It will be understood."

As this book moves forward, the next chapter will explore how artificial intelligence transforms raw data into predictive intelligence, and how learning machines become partners in healing.

Data is not replacing medicine. It is redefining it.

Chapter 8

AI & Machine Learning in Predictive Science

When Machines Learn to Anticipate Life

Artificial intelligence did not enter medicine as a sudden revolution. It arrived quietly, first as statistical tools, then as pattern recognizers, and eventually as learning systems capable of extracting meaning from complexity. In predictive science, AI and machine learning are not merely computational aids; they are the engines that transform raw biological signals into foresight. They allow medicine to move beyond observation into anticipation, beyond diagnosis into prediction.

The human body generates signals at a scale and complexity far beyond unaided human cognition. Millions of data points accumulate across time, contexts, and conditions. Within this complexity lie patterns that signal health, risk, and resilience. AI exists precisely for this purpose: to find structure where human perception sees noise, to learn relationships where linear reasoning fails, and to anticipate outcomes where certainty is impossible.

"Intelligence is not knowing the answer. It is recognizing the pattern before the answer appears."

Learning From Patterns, Not Rules

Traditional medical decision-making has relied heavily on rules and thresholds. A value crosses a predefined limit, and disease is declared.

This approach, while practical, assumes that biology behaves uniformly across individuals. It overlooks the fact that health is deeply personal and dynamic. AI and machine learning challenge this assumption by learning directly from data rather than relying on fixed rules.

Machine learning systems learn patterns through exposure. They observe examples of healthy and diseased states, identifying subtle differences in signals that correlate with future outcomes. These differences are often too complex for manual interpretation. Nonlinear interactions, temporal dependencies, and multidimensional correlations define biological systems. AI thrives in such environments.

In predictive science, learning does not stop once a model is trained. Continuous data streams allow models to update, refine, and personalize predictions. A system learns what is normal for an individual and detects deviations unique to that person. This personalization represents a fundamental shift from population-based medicine to individual-based foresight.

Importantly, machine learning models operate probabilistically. They do not predict with certainty; they estimate likelihood. This aligns with biological reality, where outcomes are shaped by interacting factors rather than deterministic rules. Prediction becomes a tool for guidance rather than a declaration of fate.

"Biology does not follow certainty. It follows probability."

From Intelligence to Foresight

Artificial intelligence becomes truly transformative when it moves beyond classification into prediction. Predictive models do not ask whether disease exists today, but how likely it is to emerge tomorrow. They analyze trajectories rather than snapshots, trends rather than thresholds.

Time-series modeling lies at the heart of predictive science. Physiological signals evolve continuously. AI systems learn how these signals change over time and how deviations correlate with future outcomes. Recurrent neural networks, deep learning architectures, and adaptive models capture temporal dependencies that static models cannot.

Speech analysis systems detect subtle changes in articulation and rhythm that precede neurological disease. Pulse waveform analysis reveals cardiovascular risk long before symptoms appear. Behavioral models identify mental health decline before emotional crisis. These capabilities emerge not from explicit programming, but from learned representation.

As predictive models mature, they increasingly integrate multiple modalities. A single signal rarely tells the full story. AI systems combine speech, pulse, movement, sleep, biochemical markers, and environmental data into unified predictions. This multimodal intelligence mirrors the holistic perspective of ancient medicine, now enhanced by computational scale.

"The future is not hidden in one signal, but revealed in their conversation."

The Emergence of Predictive Creativity

One of the most intriguing developments in AI-driven predictive science is the emergence of what may be called predictive creativity. Modern AI systems do not merely analyze existing data; they simulate possibilities. Through generative models, synthetic data, and digital twins, AI explores futures that have not yet occurred.

These capabilities allow researchers to test scenarios safely. How might disease progress under different interventions? How does lifestyle change alter risk trajectory? What happens if treatment is delayed or advanced? AI can simulate these possibilities, offering insight without experimentation on living bodies.

This creative aspect of prediction transforms medicine into a design discipline. Health becomes something that can be shaped intentionally rather than defended reactively. Physicians, researchers, and individuals collaborate with intelligent systems to design healthier futures.

The implications extend beyond individual care. Public health planning, epidemic forecasting, resource allocation, and preventive strategies can be simulated before implementation. AI becomes a tool not only for prediction, but for collective foresight.

"To predict is to imagine responsibly."

Human-AI Partnership in Healing

Despite its power, AI is not a replacement for human judgment. Predictive science does not seek to automate medicine, but to augment it. The most effective systems are those that work in partnership with clinicians, researchers, and individuals.

Human expertise provides context, ethics, empathy, and interpretation. AI provides scale, pattern recognition, and simulation. Together, they form a complementary intelligence greater than either alone. This partnership preserves the human essence of medicine while extending its reach.

Transparency and interpretability remain critical. Predictive systems must explain not only what they predict, but why. Trust emerges from understanding. As AI becomes more integrated into healthcare, ensuring that predictions are interpretable and actionable will be as important as accuracy itself.

"Technology earns trust not by being powerful, but by being understandable."

A Glimpse Into the Predictive Future

Looking ahead, AI-driven predictive science will redefine healthcare across all levels. Personalized health companions will guide daily decisions subtly and intelligently. Physicians will consult predictive dashboards that simulate outcomes before choosing interventions. Hospitals will operate as anticipatory systems rather than emergency responders. Public health strategies will be informed by forecasts rather than reaction.

Disease will not disappear. But surprise will. Fear will diminish as understanding grows. Healthcare will shift from crisis management to life stewardship.

In this future, AI does not replace the healer.

It becomes the listener. It listens to the body, the data, and the future.

"When machines learn to listen, humanity learns to live better."

As this book continues, the next chapters will explore how biomarkers give AI its language, how optimization algorithms refine prediction, and how predictive science can be deployed ethically and equitably across societies.

Artificial intelligence is not the future of medicine.

It is the instrument through which the future becomes visible.

SECTION II

Biomarkers: The Language of Disease

Chapter 9

Understanding Biomarkers: The Signatures of Life

How the Body Leaves Clues About Its Future

Every living system leaves traces of its internal state. Just as a fingerprint uniquely identifies an individual, the human body continuously produces biological signatures that reveal its condition, resilience, and vulnerability. These signatures are known as biomarkers. They are not inventions of modern science; they are discoveries—patterns that have always existed, waiting to be recognized, interpreted, and understood.

In predictive science, biomarkers are the language through which the body communicates its present and its future. They are the measurable expressions of complex biological processes, translating invisible molecular and physiological activity into signals that can be observed, quantified, and predicted. To understand biomarkers is to understand how life announces change long before it becomes visible.

"The body never hides the truth. It only speaks in a language we must learn to read."

What Biomarkers Truly Represent

A biomarker is often described as a measurable indicator of a biological state. While this definition is technically correct, it barely captures the depth of meaning biomarkers hold in predictive healthcare. A biomarker is not merely a value or a test result. It is a reflection of how the body is adapting—or failing to adapt—to internal and external demands.

At the molecular level, biomarkers reflect biochemical reactions, gene expression, protein synthesis, and cellular signaling. At the physiological level, they reflect organ function, neural regulation, and systemic balance. At the behavioral level, they reflect cognition, emotion, and interaction with the environment. Together, these layers form a continuous narrative of health.

What makes biomarkers powerful is not their ability to confirm disease, but their ability to signal deviation. Long before disease meets clinical criteria, biomarkers begin to drift. Glucose regulation becomes slightly inefficient. Neural signaling loses subtle coordination. Inflammatory markers rise quietly. Pulse variability decreases. Speech rhythm changes. These changes are often too small to trigger alarm, yet they are meaningful when interpreted in context.

Ancient physicians sensed these deviations intuitively. Modern predictive science formalizes them quantitatively. The transition from intuition to instrumentation does not diminish the value of biomarkers; it amplifies it. It allows subtle biological whispers to be heard clearly and consistently.

"Disease does not arrive suddenly. It announces itself slowly, through markers we often ignore."

Biomarkers as Predictors, Not Confirmations

Traditional medicine has largely used biomarkers as tools of confirmation. A value exceeds a threshold, and disease is diagnosed. Cholesterol crosses a limit. Blood pressure rises beyond a range. Tumor markers become elevated. These approaches are effective for identifying established disease, but they are poorly suited for prevention.

Predictive science redefines the role of biomarkers. Instead of asking whether a biomarker indicates disease today, it asks how the biomarker is changing over time and what that change implies for the future. A single measurement becomes less important than the trajectory it forms across weeks, months, and years.

This temporal perspective is critical. Two individuals may share identical biomarker values at a given moment, yet their futures may differ dramatically based on how those values arrived and where they are heading. Predictive biomarkers reveal risk by capturing trends, variability, and relationships rather than isolated points.

Modern analytics allow biomarkers to be combined into predictive signatures. A single marker may be ambiguous, but a constellation of markers tells a clearer story. Slight inflammation combined with reduced heart rate variability and altered sleep patterns may predict cardiovascular risk. Subtle speech changes combined with gait variability and micro-tremors may signal early neurodegeneration. Predictive power emerges from integration.

In this sense, biomarkers function like letters in a sentence. Individually, they convey little meaning. Together, they form language.

"A single biomarker is a word. Prediction is the sentence it completes."

The Expanding Universe of Biomarkers

The modern era has dramatically expanded the scope of what qualifies as a biomarker. Biomarkers are no longer confined to blood tests or imaging results. Advances in sensing, computation, and data science have revealed that almost any consistent biological signal can serve as a marker of health.

Speech has emerged as a powerful biomarker, carrying information about neurological integrity, emotional state, and cognitive function.

Pulse signals reveal cardiovascular and autonomic balance. Gait and movement patterns reflect neuromuscular coordination and brain health. Sleep architecture reveals metabolic and psychological resilience. Even facial expressions, eye movements, and typing patterns can signal subtle neurological or emotional changes.

This expansion aligns closely with ancient holistic medicine, which considered the entire human being as diagnostic input. The difference today lies in scale and precision. What once required years of training and subjective interpretation can now be measured continuously and analyzed objectively.

Artificial intelligence plays a central role in this transformation. AI systems learn which biomarkers matter most for specific outcomes, how they interact, and how their predictive value evolves over time. This learning process is dynamic. As new data emerges, predictive models adapt, refining their understanding of biological signatures.

Importantly, biomarkers are not static across individuals. Genetic variation, lifestyle, environment, and culture shape biomarker expression. Predictive systems must therefore learn personalized baselines. A biomarker is meaningful only in relation to the individual it represents.

"The same signal can tell different stories, depending on who is listening."

Biomarkers and the Ethics of Knowing

As biomarkers become more predictive, ethical considerations deepen. Knowing future risk carries responsibility. Information must empower, not burden. Predictive biomarkers should guide choices, not dictate outcomes. The communication of risk must be thoughtful, contextual, and compassionate.

Predictive science must also guard against reductionism. Biomarkers do not define a person. They describe tendencies, not destinies. A predicted risk does not eliminate free will; it enhances it by enabling informed decisions. The purpose of biomarkers is not to label, but to guide.

Privacy is equally critical. Biomarker data is deeply personal. As data becomes medicine, protecting it becomes a moral obligation. Trust is foundational. Without it, predictive systems cannot fulfill their promise.

"Prediction without responsibility is not progress."

The Future Written in Signatures

As this book continues, individual chapters will explore specific classes of biomarkers in greater depth—pulse, speech, neural signals, molecular markers, and behavioral patterns. Each will reveal how the body leaves signatures of its internal state and future trajectory.

Biomarkers are not merely tools of medicine. They are expressions of life itself. They reveal how the body negotiates balance, responds to stress, and adapts over time. They remind us that health is not hidden. It is written continuously within us, waiting to be read.

Predictive science does not invent this language.

It learns to listen.

"The future of health is already present, written quietly in the signatures of life."

Chapter 10

Pulse Biomarkers and Hemodynamic Patterns

Where Circulation Becomes Prediction

The pulse is the most accessible and continuous signal produced by the human body, yet it is among the most complex. What appears as a simple rhythmic beat is, in reality, a dynamic hemodynamic waveform shaped by cardiac mechanics, vascular elasticity, neural regulation, blood rheology, and systemic metabolic demand. Embedded within this waveform is a wealth of information—information that extends far beyond heart rate and reaches into the future of cardiovascular, neurological, and systemic health.

Pulse biomarkers represent one of the most promising frontiers in predictive science because they combine three rare qualities: physiological depth, non-invasive accessibility, and continuous measurability. Unlike molecular biomarkers that require laboratory intervention, pulse biomarkers can be captured effortlessly, repeatedly, and contextually. This makes them uniquely suited for longitudinal prediction rather than episodic diagnosis.

"The pulse is not a beat to be counted, but a waveform to be understood."

The Hemodynamic Language of the Pulse

Every pulse waveform is a story written in pressure and time. As the heart contracts, blood is propelled through elastic arteries, generating a pressure wave that travels, reflects, and reshapes itself as it encounters branching vessels and peripheral resistance. The resulting waveform carries information about cardiac output, arterial stiffness, vascular tone, and autonomic regulation.

In healthy systems, this waveform exhibits complexity, adaptability, and variability. Subtle changes in posture, respiration, emotion, or activity are mirrored almost instantly in pulse morphology. This responsiveness reflects physiological intelligence—the ability of the cardiovascular system to adapt continuously.

Disease alters this language. Arterial stiffness accelerates pulse wave velocity. Endothelial dysfunction dampens waveform complexity. Autonomic imbalance reduces variability. Microvascular impairment distorts reflection patterns. These changes emerge gradually, often years before overt pathology becomes clinically visible.

Traditional medicine has largely ignored these nuances, reducing the pulse to beats per minute and systolic-diastolic values. Predictive science reverses this reductionism. It treats the pulse waveform as a multidimensional signal whose shape, timing, variability, symmetry, and frequency composition carry predictive meaning.

Modern hemodynamic analysis now allows extraction of features such as waveform entropy, pulse transit time, augmentation index, reflection coefficients, and nonlinear variability measures. Each feature acts as a biomarker, revealing a different aspect of cardiovascular health. Together, they form a predictive signature far richer than any single metric.

"When variability disappears, disease is already on its way."

Pulse Biomarkers as Early Predictors of Systemic Disease

The predictive power of pulse biomarkers extends well beyond cardiovascular disorders. Because circulation is intimately connected to every organ system, hemodynamic changes often reflect systemic dysfunction.

In neurodegenerative diseases, altered autonomic regulation affects pulse variability long before motor symptoms appear. In metabolic disorders, insulin resistance and endothelial dysfunction subtly reshape pulse waveforms. In inflammatory states, vascular tone changes alter waveform morphology. Even psychological stress leaves measurable signatures in pulse dynamics through autonomic modulation.

This systemic sensitivity makes pulse biomarkers uniquely valuable for early prediction. Rather than targeting a single disease, pulse analysis reveals the body's overall resilience and regulatory capacity. Declining adaptability becomes visible as reduced variability, increased rigidity, and loss of complexity.

Recent research increasingly supports this view. Studies demonstrate that reduced heart rate variability predicts mortality across multiple conditions. Changes in pulse wave velocity predict cardiovascular risk independent of traditional factors. Nonlinear pulse dynamics correlate with aging, frailty, and cognitive decline.

Yet these findings represent only the beginning. Most current studies rely on limited datasets, short observation windows, and population averages. Predictive science demands a deeper approach—one that tracks individual pulse signatures across years, contexts, and life stages.

This opens a vast research landscape. Longitudinal pulse datasets, captured through wearable sensors, offer the opportunity to model disease trajectories rather than disease states. Machine learning systems can identify personalized pulse baselines and detect deviations unique to each individual. Digital twins can simulate how pulse dynamics evolve under different conditions.

"The pulse does not predict disease by what it is, but by how it changes."

Future Research Directions in Pulse-Based Prediction

The future of pulse biomarker research lies at the intersection of physiology, data science, and computational intelligence. One promising direction involves multimodal integration. Pulse signals gain predictive strength when combined with respiration, speech, movement, and biochemical data. Understanding how these signals interact may reveal unified biomarkers of systemic health.

Another critical direction is explainable artificial intelligence. While deep learning models can predict risk with high accuracy, understanding why a prediction was made is essential for clinical trust. Research into interpretable pulse features and transparent models will define the next generation of predictive tools.

Personalization remains central. Future research must move beyond population thresholds toward individualized prediction. This requires adaptive models that learn continuously from each person's data, adjusting predictions as physiology evolves.

There is also a need to bridge ancient pulse wisdom with modern science. Concepts such as rhythm quality, depth, and balance—long emphasized in traditional medicine—may find quantitative equivalents in waveform morphology and variability metrics. Translating these qualitative insights into measurable features could enrich predictive models and restore holistic understanding.

Finally, ethical research frameworks must evolve alongside technology. Continuous pulse monitoring generates intimate physiological narratives. Responsible data governance, consent, and patient-centered design are not optional; they are foundational.

"The future of pulse research is not faster measurement, but deeper understanding."

Toward a Predictive Circulatory Intelligence

Pulse biomarkers and hemodynamic patterns represent more than a diagnostic tool; they represent a philosophy of listening. The circulatory system is not merely a transport network. It is a sensing system, reflecting internal state and external demand continuously. Predictive science elevates this perspective, treating circulation as an intelligent communicator rather than a mechanical pump.

As pulse analysis becomes more sophisticated, it will move from clinics to daily life. Wearables will not merely count heartbeats; they will interpret waveform intelligence. Health alerts will be based not on crisis thresholds, but on trajectory deviations. Intervention will begin while the system is still adaptable.

In this future, the pulse becomes a guardian signal—a quiet companion that watches over health long before illness arrives. It reconnects modern medicine with its ancient roots, while extending predictive power far beyond what intuition alone could achieve.

The pulse has always spoken.

Only now are we learning to understand its future tense.

"To study the pulse is to study time itself, flowing through the body."

Chapter 11

Speech as a Biomarker

When the Voice Reveals the Mind and the Body

Speech is one of the most natural human behaviors. We speak without thinking, often unaware that every word we utter carries more than meaning. Embedded within speech are subtle patterns of rhythm, timing, pitch, articulation, and variability that reflect the integrity of the nervous system, the state of cognition, emotional balance, respiratory coordination, and even metabolic health. Long before disease announces itself through visible symptoms, it quietly alters the way we speak.

In predictive science, speech is emerging as one of the most powerful and accessible biomarkers. Unlike blood tests or imaging, speech requires no invasion, no specialized equipment, and no disruption of daily life. It can be captured effortlessly through ordinary devices, analyzed continuously, and interpreted remotely. Most importantly, speech reflects the functioning of multiple systems simultaneously, making it uniquely suited for early disease prediction.

"The voice does not merely express thought; it exposes the condition of the system that generates it."

The Biological Foundations of Speech

Speech is not produced by a single organ. It is the result of a finely coordinated interaction between the brain, nerves, muscles, respiratory system, and auditory feedback mechanisms. Neural circuits plan linguistic content, motor cortex regions execute articulation, cranial nerves control facial and laryngeal muscles, lungs regulate airflow, and auditory systems provide real-time correction. This complexity makes speech exquisitely sensitive to disruption.

Even minor neurological dysfunction alters timing, precision, or coordination within this system. Changes may be imperceptible to casual listeners, yet measurable through acoustic analysis. Slowed articulation, reduced pitch variability, altered pauses, tremor in voice, breathiness, and monotonic speech are not merely stylistic variations; they are physiological signals.

From a predictive standpoint, speech is valuable precisely because it is a **composite biomarker**. It reflects motor control, cognitive planning, emotional state, and autonomic regulation simultaneously. A single speech sample contains hundreds of measurable features that together form a multidimensional signature of health.

Ancient physicians recognized this intuitively. Changes in voice were noted as indicators of internal imbalance. Hoarseness, slurring, reduced clarity, and altered cadence were observed long before modern neurology existed. Today, predictive science provides the tools to quantify what intuition once sensed.

"Speech is movement made audible."

Speech and Neurological Disease Prediction

Among all applications of speech biomarkers, neurological disease prediction stands as the most advanced and promising. Disorders such as Parkinson's disease, Alzheimer's disease, amyotrophic lateral sclerosis, and other neurodegenerative conditions affect neural control of speech early in their progression.

In Parkinson's disease, for example, changes in speech often appear years before classical motor symptoms such as tremor or rigidity. Reduced vocal intensity, monotonic pitch, imprecise articulation, and altered speech rhythm reflect early dysfunction in motor planning and execution. These changes are subtle and often dismissed as aging or stress. Yet when analyzed computationally, they form a distinct predictive signature.

Research demonstrates that acoustic features such as jitter, shimmer, harmonics-to-noise ratio, formant variability, and temporal irregularities can differentiate early Parkinson's patients from healthy individuals with remarkable accuracy. Importantly, these features evolve gradually, making them suitable for longitudinal tracking and risk prediction rather than mere classification.

Cognitive disorders also leave their mark on speech. Early Alzheimer's disease and mild cognitive impairment alter language structure, word retrieval, pause patterns, and narrative coherence. Speech becomes less complex, more repetitive, and less adaptive. These changes reflect underlying neural network degradation long before memory complaints become severe.

Predictive models trained on speech data can detect these early deviations, offering the possibility of intervention at a stage when cognitive decline may still be slowed. This represents a profound shift from diagnosis after damage to prediction before irreversible loss.

"The brain begins to reveal its future through speech long before the hands begin to tremble."

Speech as a Window Into Mental and Systemic Health

Speech is not only a neurological biomarker. It is deeply influenced by emotional and physiological states. Depression, anxiety, stress disorders, and fatigue all alter speech patterns. Reduced energy, slowed tempo, flattened intonation, and increased pauses are common features of depressive speech. Anxiety introduces irregular pacing, pitch instability, and breath control issues. Chronic stress alters autonomic regulation, subtly reshaping vocal characteristics.

Predictive science leverages these changes to anticipate mental health deterioration before crisis occurs. Speech-based monitoring can identify early warning signs of emotional dysregulation, allowing timely support rather than emergency intervention. This capability is particularly valuable in populations where mental health stigma or limited access to care delays diagnosis.

Beyond mental health, speech reflects systemic conditions. Respiratory disorders alter breath control and phrasing. Cardiovascular dysfunction affects oxygenation and vocal stamina. Metabolic imbalances influence neuromuscular coordination. Even dehydration and inflammation can subtly affect voice quality. Speech, therefore, becomes a holistic biomarker, reflecting the integrated state of the body.

What makes speech uniquely powerful is its **ecological validity**. Unlike controlled laboratory tests, speech occurs naturally in daily life. It captures health in real contexts rather than artificial settings. Predictive models trained on real-world speech are therefore more robust and relevant.

"Speech carries the fingerprints of the entire organism."

From Acoustic Features to Predictive Intelligence

The transformation of speech into a predictive biomarker depends on signal processing and artificial intelligence. Raw audio signals are converted into acoustic features that capture frequency, amplitude, timing, and spectral characteristics. These features describe how speech is produced rather than what is said, preserving privacy while extracting physiological information.

Machine learning models learn patterns across these features, identifying combinations that correlate with future disease risk. Importantly, predictive models focus on change over time rather than static differences. A gradual shift in speech characteristics may be more predictive than a single abnormal sample.

Deep learning architectures further enhance this capability by learning representations directly from raw audio. These models capture complex patterns without explicit feature engineering, uncovering predictive markers that may not align with traditional linguistic categories. While powerful, these models also raise challenges related to interpretability and trust, driving research into explainable speech-based prediction.

A critical research direction lies in personalization. Speech varies widely across individuals due to language, culture, accent, and personality. Predictive systems must learn individual baselines and track deviation rather than rely on population norms. This aligns with the broader philosophy of predictive science: prediction must be personal to be meaningful.

Another promising direction involves multimodal fusion. Speech gains predictive power when combined with pulse, movement, facial expression, and physiological data. Integrated models capture interactions across systems, reflecting the holistic nature of disease progression.

"The future of speech analysis lies not in louder algorithms, but in deeper listening."

Ethical, Practical, and Future Perspectives

As speech becomes a medical biomarker, ethical considerations become paramount. Voice is deeply personal. Predictive systems must ensure privacy, consent, and transparency. The purpose of speech analysis is not surveillance, but support. Individuals must retain control over how their data is used and interpreted.

There is also a philosophical dimension. Speech-based prediction challenges the boundary between health and identity. Changes in speech are often interpreted socially rather than medically. Predictive science must navigate this sensitivity carefully, avoiding stigmatization while offering insight.

Looking ahead, speech-based biomarkers are likely to become integral to everyday healthcare. Smartphones, home assistants, and telemedicine platforms will serve as passive listeners, monitoring health unobtrusively. Early warning systems will alert individuals and clinicians to risk trajectories long before symptoms demand attention.

In research, speech datasets will expand across languages, cultures, and conditions. Models will become more inclusive, robust, and interpretable. Speech will not replace other biomarkers, but it will complement them powerfully, adding a human-centered dimension to predictive science.

Speech is universal. It is effortless. It is continuous. And it is deeply revealing.

"Before disease silences the body, it alters the voice."

Predictive science does not teach us to speak differently.

It teaches us to listen more carefully.

Chapter 12

Blood-Based and Molecular Biomarkers

The Chemical Language of the Future Written in Blood

Blood has always been regarded as the essence of life. Across civilizations, it symbolized vitality, continuity, and identity. Ancient healers observed its color, thickness, and flow to infer health, long before microscopes revealed its hidden complexity. Today, blood stands at the center of predictive science not because of symbolism, but because it is one of the most information-dense biological fluids in the human body.

Every drop of blood carries a molecular record of what the body has experienced and what it is becoming. It transports oxygen and nutrients, but it also carries hormones, immune signals, metabolic byproducts, genetic fragments, proteins, and inflammatory mediators. These molecular components fluctuate continuously in response to internal regulation and external stress. Long before disease alters organs or behavior, it reshapes this molecular landscape.

Blood-based and molecular biomarkers represent the deepest layer of predictive insight. They reveal changes that occur at the biochemical and cellular level—often years before physiological dysfunction becomes apparent. In predictive science, these biomarkers serve as early messengers, signaling future disease risk while intervention is still possible.

"Before disease changes the body, it changes the chemistry."

Molecules as Messengers of Health and Disease

At its core, disease is a molecular process. Cells alter gene expression. Proteins misfold or overexpress. Metabolic pathways shift. Immune responses become dysregulated. These changes leave measurable traces in blood long before structural damage occurs.

Glucose, lipids, inflammatory proteins, enzymes, and hormones are among the most familiar blood-based markers. Traditionally, they have been used to confirm disease after thresholds are crossed. Predictive science reinterprets these molecules not as static values, but as dynamic signals whose trajectories reveal future risk.

For example, glucose dysregulation begins subtly. Long before fasting glucose reaches diagnostic criteria for diabetes, insulin sensitivity declines and post-meal glucose variability increases. Inflammatory markers may rise intermittently, reflecting metabolic stress. Lipid profiles shift gradually, signaling vascular risk before plaque formation. These molecular drifts are predictive, not diagnostic.

Beyond traditional markers, modern molecular science has expanded the biomarker universe dramatically. Circulating microRNAs reflect gene regulation patterns. Cell-free DNA fragments reveal tissue stress and cell turnover. Proteomic signatures capture changes in protein networks. Metabolomics profiles reveal shifts in energy utilization and cellular health. Together, these molecular layers provide a multidimensional view of the body's internal state.

What makes molecular biomarkers particularly powerful is their sensitivity. Small changes at the molecular level can signal profound future consequences. Predictive science seeks to detect these changes early, before they cascade into irreversible damage.

"Molecules do not wait for symptoms. They move first."

From Single Markers to Molecular Signatures

One of the limitations of traditional medicine has been its reliance on isolated biomarkers. A single elevated value triggers concern; a normal value reassures. Biology, however, rarely behaves so simply. Disease emerges from networks of interactions rather than isolated failures.

Predictive science shifts focus from individual markers to **molecular signatures**—patterns formed by multiple biomarkers interacting over time. A single inflammatory marker may be nonspecific. Combined with metabolic indicators, hormonal shifts, and genetic predisposition, it becomes meaningful.

Artificial intelligence plays a central role in uncovering these signatures. Machine learning models analyze high-dimensional molecular data, identifying combinations that predict disease risk more accurately than any single marker. These models learn which molecules reveal early deviation and how their relationships evolve as disease progresses.

This approach has already shown promise in cancer prediction, where circulating tumor DNA and proteomic signatures can signal malignancy before imaging detects tumors. In cardiovascular disease, combined lipid, inflammatory, and metabolic signatures predict events more accurately than cholesterol alone. In neurodegeneration, molecular changes in blood reflect early neural stress long before cognitive decline becomes evident.

Predictive molecular medicine thus transforms blood tests from snapshots into timelines. The question shifts from "Is disease present?" to "Where is the body heading?"

"The future is written not in one molecule, but in the pattern they form together."

Genomics, Epigenetics, and Predictive Potential

Genetic information adds another powerful dimension to molecular biomarkers. DNA sequence reveals predisposition—risk encoded at birth. Yet genes alone do not determine destiny. Environment, behavior, and stress influence how genes are expressed. This dynamic regulation is captured through epigenetic biomarkers.

Epigenetic markers, such as DNA methylation patterns and histone modifications, reflect how life experiences shape gene activity. They change over time, responding to diet, stress, exposure, and aging. Predictive science uses these markers to estimate biological age, disease susceptibility, and resilience.

For example, accelerated epigenetic aging predicts cardiovascular disease, cognitive decline, and mortality more accurately than chronological age. Changes in gene expression patterns reveal immune dysfunction and cancer risk. These molecular clocks offer a glimpse into the body's future trajectory.

Importantly, epigenetic changes are often reversible. This makes them especially valuable for prevention. When predictive models identify epigenetic drift, lifestyle and therapeutic interventions can be guided to restore healthier patterns.

> *"Genes load the gun. Environment pulls the trigger. Prediction learns when it may fire."*

Challenges and the Path Forward

Despite their power, molecular biomarkers present challenges. High-dimensional data is complex. Interpretation requires advanced analytics. Variability across individuals complicates standardization. Ethical concerns arise around genetic and molecular privacy.

Predictive science addresses these challenges through integration and context. Molecular data gains meaning when combined with physiological, behavioral, and environmental signals. Blood-based biomarkers are not used in isolation, but as part of a holistic predictive framework.

Future research will focus on longitudinal molecular monitoring rather than episodic testing. Wearable and minimally invasive technologies may soon allow continuous biochemical sensing. AI-driven platforms will translate molecular trends into actionable insight rather than overwhelming data.

Equally important is accessibility. Molecular predictive tools must be designed not only for advanced laboratories, but for global healthcare systems. Cost-effective assays, robust models, and ethical governance will determine whether predictive molecular medicine benefits humanity broadly or remains confined to privileged settings.

"The promise of molecular prediction lies not in complexity, but in accessibility."

Blood as a Window Into the Future

Blood-based and molecular biomarkers offer the deepest glimpse into the origins of disease. They reveal how life responds at the smallest scales, how balance is lost quietly, and how intervention can restore harmony if applied early.

Predictive science does not reduce humans to molecules. It recognizes molecules as messengers—signals that, when interpreted wisely, allow us to protect life before it breaks down.

As this book continues, the next chapters will explore how neural signals, cardiac rhythms, and metabolic patterns interact with molecular biomarkers to form a unified predictive picture of health.

The future of medicine will not wait for disease to appear.

It will read the blood, listen to its signals, and act in time.

"The blood remembers the future before the body feels it."

Chapter 13

Neural and Brain-Signal Biomarkers

When the Brain Reveals the Future Before It Feels the Present

The human brain is often described as the most complex structure known to science. Composed of billions of neurons communicating through electrical and chemical signals, it governs thought, movement, emotion, memory, perception, and behavior. Yet for all its complexity, the brain leaves traces of its internal state in patterns that can be measured, analyzed, and interpreted. These patterns—neural and brain-signal biomarkers—form one of the most powerful foundations of predictive science.

Neural biomarkers do not announce disease abruptly. They evolve quietly, altering rhythm, synchronization, and signal complexity long before structural damage becomes visible. In this subtlety lies their power. By the time cognitive decline, seizures, paralysis, or psychiatric symptoms become clinically apparent, the brain's signaling patterns have often been drifting for years. Predictive science seeks to identify these drifts early, when intervention can still preserve function.

"The brain does not fail suddenly. It loses rhythm before it loses function."

The Language of Neural Signals

Neural communication is fundamentally electrical. Neurons transmit information through action potentials and synchronized oscillations, forming rhythmic patterns across different frequency bands. These rhythms are not noise. They reflect how brain networks coordinate perception, cognition, emotion, and movement.

Electroencephalography, magnetoencephalography, functional imaging, and emerging non-invasive sensing technologies capture these rhythms at varying spatial and temporal resolutions. Each modality reveals different aspects of neural behavior, but all share a common insight: healthy brains are dynamically complex. They exhibit variability, adaptability, and flexible synchronization.

Disease alters this complexity. Neural rhythms may slow, desynchronize, or become excessively rigid. Signal entropy decreases. Network connectivity weakens or becomes abnormally synchronized. These changes occur not only in neurodegenerative diseases, but across a wide spectrum of conditions including epilepsy, depression, anxiety disorders, schizophrenia, autism spectrum disorders, attention-deficit conditions, sleep disorders, chronic pain, and even systemic inflammatory diseases.

For example, early Alzheimer's disease is associated with subtle slowing of neural rhythms and reduced connectivity in memory networks. Epilepsy reveals itself through abnormal synchronization patterns long before clinical seizures. Depression alters frontal-limbic connectivity, affecting emotional regulation. Autism spectrum conditions show distinct neural synchronization patterns related to sensory processing. Sleep disorders disrupt circadian and neural oscillatory coherence, affecting metabolic and cognitive health.

Neural biomarkers, therefore, are not disease-specific signals. They are systemic indicators of how the brain organizes information. This universality makes them especially valuable for predictive science.

"When coordination weakens, disorder follows."

From Brain Signals to Disease Prediction

The predictive value of neural biomarkers lies in their temporal sensitivity. Brain-signal changes often precede symptoms by months or years. This early emergence allows predictive models to estimate risk trajectories rather than confirm established pathology.

In neurodegenerative diseases, for instance, neural network inefficiency appears before neuron loss. Cognitive tasks may still be performed adequately, but the brain expends more effort, reflected in altered signal patterns. Over time, compensation fails, and symptoms emerge. Predictive models trained on neural signals can detect this compensatory strain early.

In psychiatric disorders, neural biomarkers reveal vulnerability rather than diagnosis. Depression, anxiety, and psychosis are not binary states. They exist along continua of neural regulation. Predictive science uses brain-signal variability, connectivity patterns, and response dynamics to identify individuals at risk before crisis occurs.

In developmental and pediatric contexts, neural biomarkers provide insight into learning disorders, attention deficits, and sensory integration issues. Early detection enables supportive interventions during critical developmental windows, when the brain remains highly plastic.

Neural biomarkers also reflect systemic disease. Chronic inflammation, metabolic dysfunction, and cardiovascular insufficiency alter cerebral perfusion and neural signaling. Brain signals thus serve as integrative markers of overall physiological health.

Artificial intelligence enables this predictive power by learning complex relationships within neural data. Machine learning models identify patterns across time, frequency, and spatial domains that human observers cannot discern. These models do not merely classify disease; they estimate **how close the system is to losing stability**.

"Prediction is not about naming disease. It is about sensing instability."

Neural Plasticity and the Possibility of Prevention

One of the most hopeful aspects of neural biomarkers is their relationship with plasticity. The brain is not static. Neural networks reorganize in response to experience, learning, therapy, and environment. Predictive science leverages this adaptability.

When neural biomarkers indicate early dysfunction, interventions can be targeted to restore balance. Cognitive training, neuromodulation, behavioral therapy, lifestyle modification, and pharmacological support can alter neural trajectories. Prediction enables timely intervention, when plasticity is greatest.

This is particularly relevant in aging populations, where preserving cognitive function matters as much as prolonging life. It is equally critical in mental health, where early support prevents long-term disability. Neural prediction transforms care from crisis response to resilience building.

Future research is increasingly focused on **closed-loop predictive systems**, where neural signals are continuously monitored and interventions are adjusted dynamically. Brain-computer interfaces, adaptive neurofeedback, and personalized stimulation protocols represent the frontier of predictive neuromedicine.

"The brain that predicts its own imbalance can learn to heal."

Ethics, Identity, and the Predictive Brain

Neural data is deeply personal. Brain signals reflect thought patterns, emotional states, and identity. Predictive science must therefore approach neural biomarkers with profound ethical responsibility. Consent, transparency, and interpretability are not optional; they are essential.

Prediction must never become surveillance. Neural biomarkers should empower individuals, not label them. Risk estimation must be communicated as possibility, not inevitability. The goal is awareness, not determinism.

At a philosophical level, neural prediction challenges traditional notions of self. If future mental states can be anticipated, what does that mean for free will? Predictive science does not remove agency; it enhances it. Knowing risk creates choice. Awareness enables preparation. Understanding replaces fear.

"The purpose of prediction is not control, but freedom."

The Future of Brain-Based Predictive Medicine

As sensing technologies improve, neural biomarkers will become more accessible. Wearable and minimally invasive devices will allow continuous brain-signal monitoring in natural environments. AI models will learn individual neural signatures, detecting deviation long before dysfunction emerges.

Healthcare will shift accordingly. Neurology and psychiatry will become predictive disciplines rather than reactive specialties. Education systems may use neural biomarkers to personalize learning support. Occupational health may use them to prevent burnout. Public health may monitor population-level neural well-being during crises.

The brain will no longer be understood only through symptoms and scans. It will be understood through signals, trajectories, and adaptability.

Neural biomarkers do not tell us who we are.

They tell us how we are changing.

"The future of the mind is written in its rhythms."

As this book progresses, the next chapter will explore how cardiac signals and neural signals interact—how heart and brain together shape prediction in health and disease.

Chapter 14

Heart-Signal & ECG Biomarkers

The Electrical Signature of Life and Longevity

The heart is often described as a pump, a mechanical engine that circulates blood to sustain life. While this description is functionally correct, it fails to capture the deeper truth. The heart is not merely mechanical; it is electrical, neurological, adaptive, and communicative. Every heartbeat is governed by a complex interplay of electrical impulses, autonomic regulation, biochemical signals, and emotional states. Embedded within this activity lies one of the richest sources of predictive information available in the human body.

Heart-signal and electrocardiographic biomarkers form the backbone of predictive cardiovascular science, yet their relevance extends far beyond the heart itself. The electrical patterns of the heart reflect systemic health, neural regulation, metabolic balance, inflammatory status, and even psychological resilience. Long before symptoms arise, the heart's signals change—quietly, persistently, and measurably.

"The heart does not simply beat. It listens, responds, and remembers."

The Electrical Language of the Heart

The heart's rhythm is orchestrated by an intrinsic electrical system that initiates, propagates, and coordinates contraction. This system responds continuously to inputs from the nervous system, endocrine signals, metabolic demand, and emotional stress. The electrocardiogram captures this activity as a waveform, translating electrical propagation into time-dependent signals.

Traditionally, ECG interpretation focused on identifying gross abnormalities: arrhythmias, ischemia, conduction blocks, or acute cardiac events. Predictive science expands this scope dramatically. It treats the ECG not as a static diagnostic snapshot, but as a dynamic signal whose fine-grained properties carry predictive meaning.

Heart rate variability, beat-to-beat fluctuations, waveform morphology, repolarization dynamics, conduction timing, and nonlinear signal characteristics reflect how well the heart adapts to internal and external demands. A healthy heart is not perfectly regular. It exhibits variability, complexity, and responsiveness. Loss of this adaptability is often the earliest sign of pathology.

Autonomic imbalance, for example, reduces heart rate variability long before clinical disease appears. Chronic inflammation alters repolarization patterns. Metabolic dysfunction subtly reshapes waveform morphology. Neurological disorders affect autonomic control, changing rhythm and variability. Psychological stress leaves a measurable imprint on cardiac electrical behavior.

The ECG, therefore, is not merely a cardiac test. It is a window into systemic regulation.

"Regularity is not health. Adaptability is."

Heart Signals as Predictors of Multisystem Disease

While heart-signal biomarkers are central to cardiovascular prediction, their reach extends into multiple disease domains. The heart operates at the intersection of circulation, neural control, metabolism, and emotion. Disturbances in any of these systems affect cardiac signals.

In metabolic disorders such as diabetes and obesity, autonomic dysfunction and vascular impairment alter heart rate variability and repolarization dynamics years before complications arise. Inflammatory diseases influence electrical conduction through cytokine-mediated effects on cardiac tissue. Renal and hepatic dysfunction alter electrolyte balance, subtly changing ECG patterns. Sleep disorders disrupt circadian regulation of heart rhythms, increasing long-term cardiovascular and cognitive risk.

Neurodegenerative and psychiatric conditions also influence cardiac signaling. Parkinson's disease, depression, anxiety, and autonomic neuropathies alter heart-brain communication. These changes are often detectable through ECG analysis before motor or psychological symptoms become pronounced.

Even infectious diseases leave cardiac signatures. Systemic infections alter autonomic balance and inflammatory tone, reshaping heart-signal patterns. Predictive models trained on ECG data have shown promise in detecting early deterioration in sepsis, respiratory illness, and post-viral syndromes.

This multisystem sensitivity positions heart-signal biomarkers as integrative indicators of overall physiological resilience rather than isolated markers of cardiac health.

"The heart reflects the condition of the whole, not just itself."

From ECG Patterns to Predictive Intelligence

The transformation of heart signals into predictive biomarkers relies on advanced signal processing and artificial intelligence. Modern ECG analysis extends beyond visual interpretation into quantitative feature extraction.

Temporal dynamics, frequency components, nonlinear measures, and morphological variations are captured and analyzed.

Machine learning models learn how these features evolve over time, identifying early deviations from individual baselines. Deep learning architectures can analyze raw ECG waveforms directly, discovering predictive patterns invisible to traditional analysis. These models have demonstrated the ability to predict arrhythmias, heart failure, sudden cardiac death, and even non-cardiac conditions with remarkable accuracy.

Importantly, predictive ECG models do not operate in isolation. They integrate with other data streams—pulse waveforms, neural signals, metabolic markers, sleep patterns, and behavioral data—to form holistic predictions. This multimodal integration reflects biological reality: disease is rarely confined to a single system.

A critical research direction lies in explainable predictive cardiology. While AI models can predict outcomes, understanding why a prediction is made is essential for clinical adoption. Interpretable features such as variability loss, waveform distortion, and conduction changes help bridge the gap between algorithmic insight and medical reasoning.

Personalization is equally important. Each individual's heart has a unique electrical signature shaped by genetics, age, fitness, and lifestyle. Predictive systems must learn these personal baselines to avoid false alarms and ensure meaningful guidance.

"Prediction becomes powerful only when it becomes personal."

The Future of Heart-Based Predictive Medicine

As wearable technologies advance, continuous heart-signal monitoring is becoming ubiquitous. Smartwatches, patches, and implantable sensors collect ECG and related signals continuously, transforming episodic measurement into lifelong observation. This shift enables early detection of subtle trends that would otherwise remain invisible.

In the future, heart-signal biomarkers will guide daily decisions. Personalized alerts will recommend rest, activity modification, stress management, or medical consultation based on trajectory rather than crisis. Physicians will consult predictive cardiac dashboards that simulate outcomes under different interventions. Public health systems will monitor population-level cardiac resilience to anticipate healthcare demand.

Heart-brain integration will become a major focus. Research increasingly recognizes that cardiac signals influence cognition and emotion through bidirectional communication. Predictive science will explore how heart-signal patterns relate to mental health, cognitive decline, and stress resilience, unifying cardiology and neuroscience.

Ethical considerations remain central. Continuous monitoring must respect autonomy and privacy. Prediction must empower rather than alarm. Heart-signal data should guide care, not dictate identity.

"The purpose of knowing the heart's future is to protect the present."

Listening to the Electrical Pulse of Life

Heart-signal and ECG biomarkers represent one of the clearest examples of predictive science in action. They demonstrate how a familiar clinical tool can be reimagined as a window into the future. The heart, long associated with emotion and intuition, now stands at the forefront of computational prediction.

It speaks not in words, but in waveforms. It predicts not through certainty, but through trend.

It warns not through pain, but through subtle change.

To listen to the heart carefully is to listen to time itself moving through the body.

"The future of health is written between heartbeats."

Chapter 15

Genomic & Epigenetic Biomarkers

The Blueprint of Risk and the Memory of Life

Every human life begins with a code. Encoded within DNA lies the blueprint that shapes development, resilience, vulnerability, and potential. Yet for much of modern history, genetics was viewed as destiny—an unchangeable script written at birth. Predictive science has radically altered this perception. Today, genes are understood not as fate, but as possibility, and epigenetics reveals how life itself edits that script continuously.

Genomic and epigenetic biomarkers represent the deepest layer of prediction in healthcare. They reveal not only inherited risk, but how environment, behavior, stress, nutrition, and time interact with biology to shape disease trajectories. These biomarkers do not merely explain *why* disease occurs; they reveal *when*, *how*, and *whether* it might occur at all.

"Genes write the opening chapter. Life writes the rest."

Genomics: Inherited Risk Without Certainty

Genomic biomarkers originate from variations in DNA sequence that influence how proteins are formed, how cells respond to stress, and how systems adapt to change. Certain genetic variants increase susceptibility to cancer, cardiovascular disease, autoimmune disorders, neurodegenerative conditions, metabolic syndromes, psychiatric illness, and rare inherited diseases. Yet the presence of a risk gene does not guarantee disease.

Predictive science reframes genomics as a **probability landscape** rather than a verdict. Genetic variants modify thresholds, alter resilience, and influence response to environmental triggers. A person may carry a genetic predisposition for diabetes, yet never develop the disease if metabolic regulation remains intact. Another may carry a modest risk but develop disease early due to lifestyle, stress, or inflammation.

This complexity is precisely why genomic biomarkers are predictive rather than diagnostic. They identify vulnerability, not outcome. They help stratify risk, guide monitoring intensity, and inform preventive strategies. In oncology, genomic markers reveal susceptibility to specific cancers and predict response to targeted therapies. In cardiology, genetic variants influence lipid metabolism, vascular integrity, and arrhythmia risk. In neurology, certain genotypes modify the trajectory of cognitive decline or neurodevelopmental disorders.

Beyond common diseases, genomics plays a crucial role in predicting rare and syndromic conditions. Early identification of inherited metabolic disorders, immunodeficiencies, and neuromuscular diseases allows intervention before irreversible damage occurs. Predictive genomics thus transforms newborn screening, pediatric care, and family medicine.

Yet genomics alone cannot explain timing. Many individuals carry risk genes without disease. This temporal mystery is solved by epigenetics.

"Genetics explains possibility. Prediction explains timing."

Epigenetics: How Life Writes on the Genome

Epigenetics refers to biochemical modifications that regulate gene expression without altering DNA sequence. These modifications—such as DNA methylation and chromatin remodeling—act as switches and dimmers, turning genes on or off in response to internal and external conditions. Epigenetic biomarkers capture the biological memory of life.

Stress, nutrition, physical activity, sleep, trauma, exposure to toxins, inflammation, and aging all leave epigenetic marks. These marks accumulate gradually, altering cellular behavior and systemic regulation. Unlike genetic variants, epigenetic changes are dynamic. They evolve over time and, importantly, they are often reversible.

Predictive science leverages epigenetic biomarkers to estimate biological age, disease susceptibility, and resilience. Epigenetic clocks, for example, measure how fast the body is aging relative to chronological time. Accelerated epigenetic aging predicts cardiovascular disease, cancer risk, immune dysfunction, cognitive decline, and mortality more accurately than age alone.

In autoimmune disorders, epigenetic dysregulation alters immune tolerance long before clinical symptoms emerge. In metabolic disease, epigenetic changes influence insulin signaling and fat metabolism. In psychiatric conditions, chronic stress reshapes gene expression in neural circuits, altering emotional regulation. In cancer, epigenetic instability precedes malignant transformation.

These insights fundamentally change prevention. If disease risk is written epigenetically, it can also be rewritten.

"The genome remembers what the mind and body have endured."

From Molecular Memory to Predictive Intervention

The true power of genomic and epigenetic biomarkers emerges when they are integrated with physiological and behavioral data. Genes may load risk, but signals determine expression. Epigenetic drift may indicate vulnerability, but lifestyle determines trajectory.

Artificial intelligence enables this integration. Predictive models combine genetic predisposition with epigenetic state, molecular markers, neural signals, pulse dynamics, and behavior. These models do not predict disease in isolation; they predict **interaction**—how inherited risk interacts with lived experience.

This integration opens new research directions. Personalized prevention strategies can be designed based on genomic risk and epigenetic state. Nutritional interventions can target gene expression pathways. Stress reduction may reverse maladaptive epigenetic marks. Exercise may restore healthy regulatory patterns. Even pharmacological interventions can be guided by epigenetic responsiveness rather than trial and error.

In oncology, epigenetic biomarkers guide early detection, risk stratification, and treatment response. In neurodegeneration, they reveal how inflammation and aging interact with genetic susceptibility. In cardiovascular disease, they link lifestyle with vascular aging. In reproductive health, epigenetics explains transgenerational risk transmission, connecting parental health to offspring outcomes.

Ethical responsibility becomes paramount at this depth. Genomic and epigenetic data touch identity, family, and future generations. Predictive science must protect autonomy, avoid determinism, and emphasize empowerment. Knowledge of risk should expand choice, not constrain it.

"Prediction must illuminate possibility, not imprison identity."

The Future of Genomic Prediction

As sequencing becomes faster and more affordable, genomic data will become a routine component of healthcare. Yet the future lies not in sequencing alone, but in interpretation over time. Epigenetic monitoring may one day be continuous, revealing how daily choices shape molecular health.

Digital twins will incorporate genomic and epigenetic layers, simulating how interventions alter long-term risk. Preventive medicine will shift from generalized advice to biologically informed guidance. Healthcare will move upstream, intervening before disease acquires momentum.

Genomic and epigenetic biomarkers complete the predictive picture. They anchor the future in the past, connecting inheritance with experience. They remind us that health is neither accidental nor predetermined, but negotiated continuously between biology and life.

The genome sets the stage.

Epigenetics writes the script. Prediction gives us the power to revise it.

"The future of health is not fixed in our genes. It is shaped by how we live with them."

Chapter 16

Metabolic & Immune Biomarkers

Where Energy, Defense, and Disease Intersect

Life depends on two continuous processes that operate silently within the body: metabolism and immunity. Metabolism governs how energy is produced, stored, and utilized. Immunity governs how the body recognizes, responds to, and remembers threats. Together, these systems determine resilience, adaptation, and vulnerability. When they function harmoniously, health is sustained. When they drift out of balance, disease emerges—often gradually and invisibly.

Metabolic and immune biomarkers occupy a central position in predictive science because they reflect the body's most fundamental negotiations with its environment. Diet, stress, infection, physical activity, sleep, toxins, and aging all leave measurable imprints on metabolic and immune pathways. Long before symptoms appear, these systems signal distress through subtle biochemical and cellular changes. Predictive science listens to these signals early, when correction is still possible.

"Disease often begins not in organs, but in disturbed energy and misguided defense."

Metabolism as a Predictor of Systemic Health

Metabolism is far more than calorie balance or weight regulation. It is the biochemical engine that fuels every cellular function. Glucose utilization, lipid metabolism, mitochondrial efficiency, and hormonal regulation together define how the body produces and distributes energy. Metabolic biomarkers capture how well this engine is functioning.

Predictive science reveals that metabolic dysfunction rarely appears suddenly. Insulin resistance develops silently. Mitochondrial efficiency declines gradually. Lipid handling becomes inefficient. These changes may occur years before diabetes, cardiovascular disease, fatty liver disease, polycystic ovarian syndrome, or obesity are diagnosed.

Subtle elevations in fasting insulin, increased glucose variability, altered lipid particle profiles, and changes in metabolic flexibility signal early imbalance. Even in individuals with "normal" laboratory values, trajectories matter. A slow upward drift, reduced adaptability to stress, or delayed recovery after metabolic challenge predicts future disease risk.

Metabolic biomarkers also extend into neurological and psychiatric domains. The brain is one of the most energy-demanding organs. Impaired glucose metabolism affects cognition, mood regulation, and neuroplasticity. Increasing evidence links metabolic dysfunction to depression, cognitive decline, and neurodegenerative disorders. In this sense, metabolic biomarkers predict not only physical disease, but mental health outcomes as well.

Cancer biology also intersects deeply with metabolism. Tumor cells rewire metabolic pathways to support uncontrolled growth. Predictive metabolic signatures may reveal early oncogenic processes before tumors become detectable through imaging.

"Energy mismanagement is one of the earliest warnings the body provides."

Immune Biomarkers and the Quiet Rise of Inflammation

The immune system is designed to protect, but its power must be precisely regulated. Acute immune responses save lives. Chronic immune activation, however, slowly damages tissues and disrupts signaling. Predictive science increasingly recognizes chronic low-grade inflammation as a common thread linking diverse diseases.

Immune biomarkers capture this state of persistent activation. Subtle elevations in inflammatory mediators, shifts in immune cell populations, and altered cytokine balance signal immune dysregulation long before autoimmune disease, cardiovascular events, metabolic syndrome, or neurodegeneration emerge.

Autoimmune disorders such as rheumatoid arthritis, lupus, multiple sclerosis, and inflammatory bowel disease often begin with years of immune imbalance before clinical symptoms appear. Predictive immune biomarkers offer a window into this preclinical phase, enabling monitoring and early modulation.

Chronic inflammation also plays a central role in cancer initiation and progression. Immune dysregulation creates a permissive environment for genetic instability and tumor growth. Predictive immune profiling may therefore identify individuals at increased oncological risk well before malignancy develops.

Infectious diseases leave immune signatures that persist beyond acute illness. Post-viral syndromes, immune exhaustion, and dysregulated immune memory alter metabolic and neurological function. Predictive monitoring of immune recovery trajectories can guide rehabilitation and prevent long-term complications.

The immune system is also deeply connected to mental health. Inflammatory signaling influences neurotransmission and stress response. Depression, anxiety, and cognitive impairment increasingly show immune correlates. Predictive immune biomarkers thus bridge physical and psychological health.

"When defense forgets how to stop, disease finds a way to begin."

Metabolic–Immune Interaction: The Predictive Core

Perhaps the most powerful insight of predictive science lies in understanding that metabolism and immunity are not separate systems. They are deeply intertwined. Immune cells depend on metabolic pathways for activation and regulation. Metabolic dysfunction alters immune behavior. Together, they form a feedback loop that amplifies or resolves disease risk.

Insulin resistance promotes inflammation. Inflammation worsens metabolic efficiency. Obesity alters immune cell composition. Immune dysregulation impairs hormonal balance. This reciprocal relationship explains why metabolic and immune biomarkers are among the earliest predictors of systemic disease.

Artificial intelligence excels at modeling these interactions. Predictive models integrate metabolic markers, immune profiles, behavioral data, and physiological signals to identify risk trajectories that would otherwise remain hidden. These models do not seek a single cause. They map networks of influence.

Future research increasingly focuses on **metabolic–immune phenotypes** rather than isolated diagnoses. Individuals may share disease labels but differ profoundly in underlying metabolic and immune dynamics. Personalized prediction allows interventions to target the dominant imbalance rather than applying generic treatment.

Lifestyle interventions gain scientific precision through this lens. Diet alters immune tone. Exercise restores metabolic flexibility. Sleep regulates inflammatory rhythms. Stress management recalibrates immune response.

Predictive biomarkers allow these interventions to be timed and tailored for maximum impact.

"Prediction is most powerful where systems meet."

Toward a Predictive Model of Resilience

Metabolic and immune biomarkers do not merely predict disease; they predict resilience. A body that maintains metabolic flexibility and immune balance adapts to stress, resists illness, and recovers efficiently. Predictive science shifts focus from pathology to capacity.

Future healthcare systems will monitor metabolic and immune signals continuously, detecting early drift and recommending corrective action. Wearable sensors, minimally invasive testing, and AI-driven analytics will translate biochemical complexity into actionable insight. Preventive care will become dynamic rather than episodic.

Ethical responsibility remains essential. Metabolic and immune data reveal vulnerability, but vulnerability is not destiny. Predictive science must emphasize empowerment, not fear. The goal is not to medicalize normal variation, but to support balance.

Metabolism tells us how the body uses energy.

Immunity tells us how the body protects itself.

Together, they tell us how long health can last.

"The future of disease prevention lies in restoring balance before damage accumulates."

As this journey continues, the next chapter will explore how vision and ocular biomarkers reveal systemic and neurological disease risk, expanding predictive science into yet another sensory dimension.

SECTION III

Predicting Specific Diseases

Chapter 17

Predicting Parkinson's Disease

Listening to the Body Long Before It Begins to Tremble

Parkinson's disease has long been understood as a disorder of movement. Tremor, rigidity, slowness, and postural instability dominate clinical descriptions and public perception. Yet these visible signs represent only the final chapter of a much longer story. Long before the hands shake or the gait changes, Parkinson's disease begins silently—altering neural rhythms, speech patterns, autonomic regulation, sensory processing, and molecular balance.

Predictive science reframes Parkinson's disease not as a sudden neurological failure, but as a slow, measurable drift across multiple biological systems. This shift in perspective is profound. It suggests that Parkinson's disease is not merely diagnosable, but **predictable**—often years before clinical recognition.

"By the time tremor appears, the disease has already been speaking for a long time."

The Long Silent Phase of Parkinson's Disease

One of the defining features of Parkinson's disease is its prolonged prodromal phase. During this period, individuals may experience subtle, non-specific changes that are rarely connected to neurological disease. Mild voice alteration, reduced facial expression, sleep disturbances, constipation, fatigue, mood changes, and reduced sense of smell often appear years before motor symptoms.

Traditional medicine treats these signs as unrelated complaints. Predictive science recognizes them as **early signals of neural system imbalance**. Parkinson's disease affects not only dopaminergic neurons, but also autonomic, sensory, and cortical networks. As a result, its earliest fingerprints appear across diverse biomarker domains.

Neural signaling patterns begin to shift subtly. Brain rhythms lose complexity. Coordination between motor and cognitive networks becomes less efficient. Autonomic regulation weakens, altering heart rate variability and gastrointestinal function. Speech articulation and vocal modulation degrade imperceptibly. These changes are gradual and adaptive at first, allowing the individual to function normally while the disease progresses quietly.

This silent phase represents the most valuable window for prediction and intervention. Once motor symptoms emerge, significant neuronal loss has already occurred. Predictive science seeks to identify Parkinson's disease while neural systems are still compensating, not after they have failed.

"Parkinson's disease does not begin with movement. It begins with miscommunication."

Biomarker Convergence in Parkinson's Prediction

No single biomarker can predict Parkinson's disease reliably. Its strength lies in convergence. Predictive accuracy emerges when multiple signals are interpreted together, revealing a coherent trajectory rather than isolated abnormalities.

Speech is one of the earliest and most accessible indicators. Even in the absence of audible impairment, acoustic analysis reveals reduced pitch variability, altered articulation timing, diminished vocal energy, and increased micro-instability. These changes reflect early motor planning and execution deficits long before speech becomes clinically impaired.

Neural and brain-signal biomarkers provide deeper insight. Altered synchronization patterns, reduced signal entropy, and inefficiencies in motor network coordination indicate early neurophysiological drift. These changes are subtle, but consistent across longitudinal measurements.

Cardiac and autonomic biomarkers add another layer. Reduced heart rate variability and altered autonomic balance reflect degeneration beyond motor pathways. Parkinson's disease affects the autonomic nervous system early, making heart-signal biomarkers valuable predictors of disease onset and progression.

Eye and vision-based biomarkers contribute additional predictive power. Abnormal eye movements, reduced blink rate, impaired visual contrast sensitivity, and altered pupil dynamics reflect dysfunction in neural circuits involved in motor control and attention. These changes often appear before motor impairment becomes evident.

Molecular and metabolic biomarkers further strengthen prediction. Inflammatory markers, oxidative stress indicators, mitochondrial dysfunction signals, and altered metabolic profiles reflect systemic involvement. While not specific on their own, they reinforce predictive models when combined with neural and behavioral signals.

Genomic and epigenetic factors modify susceptibility and progression. Certain genetic variants increase risk, while epigenetic markers reveal how aging, stress, and environment accelerate neurodegeneration. Predictive models integrate these layers to estimate individual risk trajectories rather than binary outcomes.

"Prediction emerges not from one signal,
but from harmony among many."

Artificial Intelligence and Longitudinal Prediction

The complexity of Parkinson's disease makes it an ideal candidate for artificial intelligence–driven prediction. Machine learning models excel at detecting subtle, multidimensional patterns that unfold slowly over time. Rather than searching for diagnostic thresholds, predictive systems learn **trajectories of change**.

Longitudinal data is central to this approach. A single speech sample or ECG recording offers limited insight. Continuous or periodic monitoring over months and years reveals trends—small deviations that accumulate meaning. Predictive models compare individuals not to population averages, but to their own historical baselines.

Digital twins play an increasingly important role in Parkinson's prediction. These computational models simulate how an individual's biomarkers might evolve under different conditions. They allow researchers and clinicians to explore "what-if" scenarios, evaluating how interventions such as exercise, medication, sleep optimization, or stress reduction might alter disease trajectory.

Importantly, predictive models are shifting from classification to **risk estimation**. Rather than declaring whether Parkinson's disease is present, they estimate likelihood, timing, and progression speed. This probabilistic approach aligns with biological reality and avoids false certainty.

Explainability remains crucial. Clinicians and individuals must understand why a risk estimate has changed. Transparent models that highlight contributing signals build trust and guide intervention.

"The goal is not to predict diagnosis, but to predict direction."

From Prediction to Prevention and Care

The predictive identification of Parkinson's disease opens new possibilities for care. Early-stage intervention focuses not on symptom suppression, but on **neural preservation and resilience**. Lifestyle modifications, targeted therapy, neuromodulation, and personalized rehabilitation strategies can slow progression and preserve quality of life.

Predictive monitoring also empowers individuals. Awareness of risk enables proactive planning, informed decision-making, and emotional preparedness. Importantly, prediction does not imply inevitability. Many individuals with elevated risk may never develop disabling disease if protective factors are strengthened early.

Ethical responsibility is central. Predicting neurodegenerative disease carries psychological weight. Predictive systems must prioritize informed consent, clear communication, and supportive guidance. Risk information should be framed as opportunity, not doom.

From a research perspective, predictive Parkinson's models offer unprecedented insight into disease mechanisms. Studying individuals in the prodromal phase reveals how neurodegeneration begins and spreads. This knowledge accelerates therapeutic discovery and shifts research focus from late-stage pathology to early intervention.

"To predict Parkinson's disease is not to predict decline, but to protect possibility."

A Model for Future Neurodegenerative Prediction

Parkinson's disease serves as a model for predictive neurology. Its long silent phase, multisystem involvement, and measurable early signals make it ideal for demonstrating how predictive science can transform care.

As technology advances, predictive Parkinson's monitoring may become routine. Smartphones may analyze speech daily. Wearables may track autonomic and motor signals continuously. Eye-tracking may assess neural coordination unobtrusively. Molecular assays may reveal subtle neuroinflammatory changes. AI systems will integrate these signals into coherent risk narratives.

This future does not replace clinicians. It augments them. Predictive science provides foresight; human care provides meaning.

Parkinson's disease teaches us a critical lesson:

Disease whispers before it speaks.

The future belongs to those who listen early.

"The greatest victory over disease is not treatment, but timely understanding."

Chapter 18

Predicting Alzheimer's & Cognitive Decline

When Memory Begins to Fade Long Before It Is Lost

Alzheimer's disease is often perceived as a sudden theft of memory, a gradual erasure of identity that begins only when forgetfulness becomes undeniable. In reality, cognitive decline does not begin with missed names or misplaced objects. It begins silently, years—sometimes decades—before diagnosis, as neural efficiency diminishes, metabolic balance shifts, and communication between brain networks becomes subtly impaired.

Predictive science challenges the traditional narrative of Alzheimer's disease. It reframes cognitive decline not as an inevitable consequence of aging, but as a **detectable and modifiable trajectory**. Long before memory loss interferes with daily life, the brain reveals early signals of vulnerability. These signals, when interpreted collectively, allow us to anticipate decline and intervene while cognitive resilience can still be preserved.

"Memory does not disappear suddenly. It loses precision before it loses presence."

The Invisible Onset of Cognitive Decline

One of the most striking aspects of Alzheimer's disease is its prolonged preclinical phase. During this stage, individuals appear cognitively normal by conventional testing, yet subtle inefficiencies are already emerging within neural networks. The brain compensates by recruiting additional regions to perform tasks that once required minimal effort. This compensation masks decline, but it also leaves measurable traces.

Neural signal complexity begins to diminish. Communication between memory, attention, and executive networks becomes less synchronized. Processing speed slows imperceptibly. Sleep architecture changes, reducing the brain's ability to clear metabolic waste. These shifts rarely trigger clinical concern, yet they form the earliest predictive markers of future decline.

Behavioral changes often precede memory complaints. Difficulty multitasking, reduced mental flexibility, subtle language simplification, or increased mental fatigue reflect early network strain. Emotional regulation may change as well, with increased anxiety or withdrawal emerging quietly.

Predictive science recognizes these signs not as normal aging, but as **early cognitive stress indicators**. Aging itself does not inevitably cause Alzheimer's disease. The divergence between healthy cognitive aging and pathological decline begins far earlier than previously assumed.

"The brain signals fatigue long before it admits failure."

Biomarker Pathways in Alzheimer's Prediction

Alzheimer's disease is not defined by a single pathology. It is the outcome of interacting processes involving neural degeneration, metabolic dysfunction, vascular impairment, inflammation, and impaired clearance mechanisms. Predictive accuracy emerges when these pathways are interpreted together.

Neural and brain-signal biomarkers reveal early network inefficiency. Reduced signal variability, altered oscillatory patterns, and weakened connectivity in memory-related circuits appear before structural atrophy. These changes reflect functional decline rather than neuron loss, making them ideal for early prediction.

Speech and language biomarkers provide additional insight. Subtle changes in vocabulary diversity, sentence complexity, pause patterns, and narrative coherence often emerge early. These changes are not always perceived as memory loss, yet they reflect declining cognitive integration and retrieval efficiency.

Sleep-related biomarkers are increasingly recognized as central to prediction. Impaired deep sleep disrupts the brain's glymphatic system, reducing clearance of neurotoxic proteins. Sleep fragmentation, altered circadian rhythms, and reduced slow-wave activity are predictive of future cognitive decline.

Cardiovascular and metabolic biomarkers also play a critical role. Cerebral perfusion depends on vascular health. Hypertension, insulin resistance, and metabolic syndrome impair blood flow and energy supply to neural tissue. Predictive models consistently show that metabolic and vascular dysfunction accelerate cognitive decline.

Eye and vision-based biomarkers further strengthen prediction. Retinal nerve fiber thinning, altered eye movement patterns, and impaired contrast sensitivity reflect early neural degeneration. The eye, as an extension of the brain, offers a non-invasive window into cognitive health.

Molecular and blood-based biomarkers complete the picture. Inflammatory markers, lipid dysregulation, and protein clearance inefficiencies signal systemic contributors to neurodegeneration. While classical biomarkers such as amyloid and tau have dominated Alzheimer's research, predictive science emphasizes **dynamic change and interaction**, not static presence.

Genomic and epigenetic factors modify vulnerability and progression. Certain genetic profiles increase risk, but epigenetic drift influenced by lifestyle, stress, and aging determines whether and when disease manifests.

"Cognitive decline is not caused by one failure, but by many small compromises."

Artificial Intelligence and Long-Term Cognitive Forecasting

The complexity of Alzheimer's disease makes it particularly well suited for AI-driven prediction. Machine learning systems integrate diverse data streams, learning patterns that unfold slowly over time. Rather than diagnosing Alzheimer's disease, predictive models estimate cognitive resilience, vulnerability, and rate of decline.

Longitudinal monitoring is essential. Cognitive trajectories matter more than absolute scores. Predictive systems compare individuals to their own baselines, detecting subtle deviations that accumulate meaning. A gradual decline in speech complexity, combined with altered sleep patterns and reduced neural variability, may predict risk years before diagnosis.

Digital twins represent a powerful future tool in cognitive prediction. These models simulate how an individual's brain might age under different conditions, allowing clinicians and individuals to explore intervention strategies virtually. Nutrition, exercise, sleep optimization, cognitive training, and stress reduction can be tested computationally before being applied in life.

Explainability remains crucial. Predictive systems must communicate risk in ways that are understandable and supportive. Cognitive prediction carries emotional weight, and transparency is essential to avoid fear-driven decision-making.

"Prediction does not steal certainty. It restores choice."

From Prediction to Cognitive Preservation

The ultimate goal of predicting Alzheimer's disease is not early labeling, but **early preservation**. Cognitive decline is most modifiable in its earliest stages, when neural plasticity remains intact. Interventions applied during this window can slow progression and maintain quality of life.

Lifestyle factors become powerful medicine when guided by predictive insight. Physical activity improves cerebral perfusion. Cognitive engagement strengthens network resilience. Sleep optimization restores clearance mechanisms. Metabolic control protects neural energy supply. Social connection buffers emotional and cognitive decline.

Predictive monitoring also reframes aging. Rather than fearing inevitable decline, individuals can track cognitive health proactively, responding to early warning signals with informed action. Healthcare systems shift from crisis management to cognitive longevity.

Ethical responsibility is paramount. Predictive knowledge must empower, not burden. Risk information should be framed as a dynamic probability, not a fixed destiny. Individuals must retain autonomy over how and when they engage with predictive data.

"To predict cognitive decline is not to predict loss, but to protect memory."

A New Narrative for Alzheimer's Disease

Alzheimer's disease has long been associated with helplessness and inevitability. Predictive science offers a new narrative—one of anticipation, preparation, and resilience. It teaches us that the brain speaks long before it forgets, and that listening early can change outcomes.

As predictive tools mature, Alzheimer's disease may no longer be detected only when memory is lost, but when balance begins to shift. The future of cognitive health lies not in curing disease after it appears, but in preserving function before it fades.

Memory does not vanish overnight.

It withdraws quietly. Prediction gives us the chance to call it back.

"The future of the mind depends on how early we choose to listen."

Chapter 19

Predicting Cardiovascular Disorders

When the Heart Warns Long Before It Breaks

Cardiovascular disease is often described as sudden—an unexpected heart attack, an abrupt stroke, a collapse without warning. Yet in reality, the heart almost never fails silently. It adapts, compensates, and signals distress long before catastrophe occurs. Predictive science reveals that cardiovascular disorders are not abrupt events, but **slowly evolving trajectories**, written into physiology years before symptoms demand attention.

The heart exists at the intersection of circulation, metabolism, neural regulation, and emotion. As a result, cardiovascular disease is rarely confined to the heart alone. It reflects systemic imbalance—vascular stiffness, metabolic stress, chronic inflammation, autonomic dysregulation, and behavioral strain. Predictive science listens to these interconnected signals early, when intervention can still restore balance.

"The heart does not suddenly collapse. It negotiates survival for years before it yields."

The Silent Progression of Cardiovascular Risk

A defining feature of cardiovascular disease is its long asymptomatic phase. Atherosclerosis develops quietly. Blood vessels lose elasticity gradually. Endothelial function declines slowly. The body compensates by increasing pressure, altering flow, and redistributing workload. During this time, individuals may feel healthy, even as risk accumulates beneath the surface.

Predictive science reframes this silent progression as an opportunity rather than a limitation. Subtle changes in vascular tone, pulse wave velocity, heart rate variability, and blood pressure dynamics reveal early dysfunction. These changes are not random. They follow recognizable patterns that precede clinical events by years or decades.

Metabolic imbalance accelerates this trajectory. Insulin resistance, lipid dysregulation, and visceral adiposity increase vascular inflammation and oxidative stress. Chronic low-grade inflammation weakens arterial integrity and disrupts nitric oxide signaling. Autonomic imbalance reduces cardiovascular adaptability, making the system less resilient to stress.

Psychological stress further compounds risk. Emotional strain alters autonomic tone, increases inflammatory signaling, and disrupts circadian regulation. Predictive cardiovascular models increasingly recognize stress and behavioral patterns as integral components of risk rather than secondary factors.

"Risk accumulates quietly. Prediction gives it a voice."

Biomarker Convergence in Cardiovascular Prediction

Cardiovascular prediction does not rely on a single measurement. Blood pressure alone cannot explain risk. Cholesterol alone does not predict events reliably. Predictive accuracy emerges from the **convergence of multiple biomarkers**, interpreted over time.

Pulse and hemodynamic biomarkers reveal vascular health dynamically. Increased pulse wave velocity indicates arterial stiffening. Altered waveform reflection patterns signal microvascular dysfunction. Reduced variability suggests declining adaptability. These signals often appear before structural disease is detectable.

Heart-signal and ECG biomarkers provide insight into electrical stability and autonomic regulation. Subtle repolarization changes, conduction delays, and reduced heart rate variability reflect early dysfunction in cardiac control mechanisms. These changes may precede arrhythmias, heart failure, or ischemic events.

Metabolic and immune biomarkers add another dimension. Inflammatory markers, insulin dynamics, lipid particle composition, and oxidative stress indicators reveal systemic contributors to cardiovascular disease. These markers often interact synergistically, amplifying risk when combined.

Neural biomarkers further strengthen prediction. The heart and brain are linked through bidirectional communication. Autonomic dysregulation alters cardiac behavior, while vascular insufficiency affects cognitive and emotional regulation. Predictive models increasingly integrate neural and cardiac signals to assess systemic resilience.

Eye-based biomarkers offer additional insight. Retinal microvascular changes reflect cerebral and systemic vascular health. These changes correlate strongly with future cardiovascular and cerebrovascular events, making ocular assessment a valuable predictive tool.

Genomic and epigenetic factors modify susceptibility and progression. Genetic variants influence lipid metabolism, coagulation, and vascular integrity, while epigenetic drift reflects lifestyle and environmental impact on cardiovascular aging.

"The future of the heart is written across many systems."

Artificial Intelligence and Cardiovascular Trajectories

The complexity of cardiovascular disease makes it ideally suited for artificial intelligence–driven prediction. Machine learning models analyze longitudinal data, identifying subtle interactions that escape conventional risk scoring systems. Rather than categorizing individuals as "high" or "low" risk, predictive systems estimate trajectories—how quickly risk is accumulating and how it responds to intervention.

Continuous monitoring plays a central role. Wearable devices capture heart rate dynamics, rhythm stability, activity patterns, and sleep quality. When combined with periodic biochemical and imaging data, these signals form a living cardiovascular profile.

Digital twins enable simulation of cardiovascular futures. By modeling how blood pressure control, metabolic improvement, stress reduction, or medication adherence alters trajectory, predictive systems transform prevention into a personalized strategy rather than a generic recommendation.

Explainability remains essential. Predictive insight must be interpretable, allowing clinicians and individuals to understand which factors are driving risk and how change can influence outcome. This transparency builds trust and supports sustained engagement.

"Prediction becomes meaningful only when it guides action."

From Early Warning to Cardiovascular Resilience

The ultimate goal of cardiovascular prediction is not merely event prevention, but **resilience preservation**. A resilient cardiovascular system adapts efficiently to stress, maintains vascular flexibility, and recovers quickly. Predictive science focuses on restoring this adaptability rather than chasing static targets.

Early intervention guided by prediction is often simpler and more effective than late-stage treatment. Lifestyle modification, targeted therapy, behavioral change, and stress management have the greatest impact when applied early. Predictive insight ensures these interventions are timely rather than reactive.

Ethical responsibility remains central. Predictive cardiovascular data must empower individuals, not induce anxiety. Risk should be communicated as modifiable probability, not inevitability. Autonomy and informed choice must guide all predictive care.

Cardiovascular prediction also reshapes public health. Population-level monitoring of cardiovascular resilience allows healthcare systems to anticipate demand, allocate resources proactively, and design prevention strategies tailored to community needs.

"The heart thrives not on certainty, but on adaptability."

A New Paradigm for Heart Health

Cardiovascular disease has long been treated as an emergency problem. Predictive science transforms it into a **timeline problem**—one that unfolds gradually and can be redirected early. By listening to the heart's signals across systems and time, we gain the opportunity to protect health rather than respond to crisis.

The heart speaks continuously. It signals strain, adaptation, and resilience. Prediction teaches us to listen early and act wisely.

"The greatest cardiovascular intervention is not performed in the emergency room, but years before the first event."

Chapter 20

Predicting Diabetes & Metabolic Disorders

When Energy Regulation Begins to Drift Before Disease Appears

Diabetes and metabolic disorders are often described as lifestyle diseases, conditions that emerge abruptly when blood sugar crosses a diagnostic threshold. In truth, metabolic disease rarely begins at diagnosis. It unfolds silently over years, sometimes decades, as the body's finely tuned systems for energy regulation gradually lose flexibility. Predictive science reframes diabetes not as a sudden failure of glucose control, but as a **progressive loss of metabolic adaptability**—a process that can be observed, measured, and redirected long before irreversible damage occurs.

Metabolism governs how the body converts nutrients into energy, how it stores excess fuel, and how it responds to stress and demand. When this system functions well, the body adapts effortlessly to changing conditions. When it begins to drift, subtle signals appear across multiple systems. Predictive science listens to these signals early, when restoration is still possible.

"Metabolic disease does not begin with sugar. It begins with lost flexibility."

The Long Metabolic Drift Before Diagnosis

One of the most misunderstood aspects of diabetes is its prolonged preclinical phase. Blood glucose may remain within normal limits while deeper dysfunction advances. Insulin sensitivity declines quietly. Post-meal glucose fluctuations increase. Fat metabolism becomes inefficient. Mitochondrial performance wanes. These changes often occur without noticeable symptoms, allowing disease risk to accumulate unnoticed.

Predictive science recognizes this phase as the most critical window for intervention. Subtle elevations in fasting insulin, increased glycemic variability, delayed glucose clearance, and altered lipid profiles reveal early metabolic strain. These changes are dynamic rather than static. The body may compensate temporarily, masking dysfunction until resilience is exhausted.

Chronic stress accelerates this drift. Stress hormones alter glucose regulation, promote visceral fat accumulation, and impair insulin signaling. Sleep disruption compounds the problem by altering circadian metabolic rhythms. Inflammatory signaling further disrupts insulin sensitivity, creating a self-reinforcing cycle.

Importantly, metabolic dysfunction rarely exists in isolation. It interacts with cardiovascular health, immune regulation, cognitive function, reproductive health, and even mood. Predictive models consistently show that early metabolic imbalance predicts a wide range of future disorders, not just diabetes.

"The body adapts to imbalance until adaptation itself becomes the disease."

Biomarker Pathways in Metabolic Prediction

Predicting diabetes and metabolic disorders requires a holistic view of biomarkers rather than reliance on glucose alone. Glucose levels represent an outcome, not the process. Predictive insight emerges when multiple metabolic signals are interpreted together.

Insulin dynamics provide one of the earliest indicators. Elevated insulin levels in the presence of normal glucose reveal compensatory strain. Over time, this compensation fails, leading to overt hyperglycemia. Tracking insulin sensitivity over time offers predictive power far beyond single glucose measurements.

Lipid metabolism adds another layer. Altered lipid particle size, triglyceride elevation, and impaired fatty acid oxidation reflect metabolic inflexibility. These changes often precede diabetes and strongly predict cardiovascular risk.

Inflammatory biomarkers reveal immune-metabolic interaction. Low-grade chronic inflammation interferes with insulin signaling and mitochondrial function. Predictive models show that inflammation often precedes metabolic breakdown rather than resulting from it.

Neural and autonomic biomarkers further enhance prediction. Reduced heart rate variability reflects impaired autonomic regulation of metabolism. The brain plays a central role in energy homeostasis, and early dysregulation in neural control can accelerate metabolic decline.

Eye and vascular biomarkers offer additional insight. Retinal microvascular changes reflect early metabolic damage, even before diabetic retinopathy develops. These changes correlate with future risk of systemic complications.

Genomic and epigenetic factors modify susceptibility. Genetic predisposition influences insulin sensitivity and fat distribution, while epigenetic drift reflects lifestyle and environmental impact. Predictive science integrates these layers to estimate individual metabolic trajectories rather than categorical diagnoses.

*"Metabolic prediction is not about numbers.
It is about patterns over time."*

Artificial Intelligence and Metabolic Trajectories

The complexity of metabolic disease makes it particularly amenable to artificial intelligence–driven prediction. Machine learning models analyze longitudinal metabolic data, identifying subtle interactions that traditional thresholds miss. Rather than waiting for diagnostic cutoffs, predictive systems track how metabolic flexibility changes over time.

Wearable technologies contribute valuable data. Continuous glucose monitoring reveals glycemic variability and response to meals. Activity trackers capture energy expenditure and circadian rhythm alignment. Sleep metrics reveal recovery efficiency. When combined, these signals form a living metabolic profile.

Digital twins enable simulation of metabolic futures. Predictive systems can model how dietary changes, physical activity, stress reduction, or medication influence long-term metabolic health. This allows individuals and clinicians to explore intervention strategies before committing to them in life.

Explainability remains essential. Predictive insights must be communicated clearly, highlighting which behaviors and physiological signals are driving risk. This transparency supports sustained engagement and avoids confusion or fear.

"Prediction empowers change only when it is understood."

Beyond Diabetes: The Metabolic Web of Disease

Predicting metabolic dysfunction extends far beyond diabetes prevention. Metabolic imbalance influences obesity, fatty liver disease, polycystic ovarian syndrome, infertility, cardiovascular disease, cognitive decline, and even certain cancers. Predictive metabolic monitoring therefore protects multiple dimensions of health simultaneously.

In women's health, early metabolic prediction informs reproductive planning and prevents long-term complications. In aging populations, preserving metabolic flexibility supports cognitive and physical resilience. In pediatric populations, early metabolic signals guide lifelong health trajectories.

Metabolic prediction also reshapes public health. Population-level monitoring of metabolic resilience enables proactive policy design, targeted intervention, and resource optimization. Rather than reacting to disease burden, healthcare systems can anticipate and reduce it.

Ethical responsibility remains central. Predictive metabolic data must empower rather than stigmatize. Body weight, glucose levels, and metabolic markers are deeply personal. Prediction should guide supportive care, not judgment.

"Metabolic health is not a moral failing.
It is a biological negotiation."

Toward a Future of Metabolic Resilience

The future of diabetes care lies not in better insulin delivery alone, but in earlier prediction and preservation of metabolic adaptability. Predictive science shifts focus from controlling disease to sustaining balance.

When metabolic drift is identified early, interventions are often simple and effective. Small adjustments in diet, movement, sleep, and stress can restore flexibility. Predictive insight ensures these changes occur before damage accumulates.

Diabetes teaches us a critical lesson about health: the body rarely fails suddenly. It signals imbalance repeatedly, patiently, waiting to be heard.

Prediction allows us to listen in time.

"The future of metabolic health is not measured in glucose, but in adaptability."

Chapter 21

Predicting Cancer & Tumor Progression

When Cells Whisper Long Before They Turn Malignant

Cancer is often experienced as a sudden rupture in life—a diagnosis that arrives unexpectedly, carrying fear, urgency, and uncertainty. Yet cancer, like most chronic diseases, does not arise overnight. It is the end result of a prolonged biological conversation, unfolding quietly within cells and tissues long before a tumor becomes visible or symptoms emerge. Predictive science invites us to listen to this conversation early, when the language of disease is still subtle and intervention can change its course.

At its core, cancer is a disorder of regulation. Cells lose their ability to respond appropriately to signals that govern growth, repair, and death. This loss does not occur abruptly. It is preceded by years of molecular instability, immune evasion, metabolic rewiring, and microenvironmental change. Predictive science reframes cancer not merely as a disease to be detected, but as a **trajectory to be anticipated and redirected**.

"Cancer does not announce itself.
It negotiates silently with the body for years."

The Long Prelude to Malignancy

Before a tumor forms, cells pass through intermediate states of vulnerability. DNA repair mechanisms become less efficient. Epigenetic regulation drifts. Inflammatory signaling increases. Metabolic pathways are subtly altered to support survival under stress. These changes often coexist without producing immediate harm, allowing the body to compensate and maintain apparent health.

Predictive science focuses on this preclinical phase, where instability accumulates but transformation is not yet complete. Genomic mutations may appear sporadically, but it is the surrounding environment that determines whether they persist or are eliminated. Chronic inflammation creates a permissive context for mutation. Metabolic stress favors abnormal growth strategies. Immune surveillance weakens gradually, allowing aberrant cells to escape detection.

These early changes are measurable. Circulating molecular fragments, altered metabolic profiles, immune imbalance, and epigenetic drift all signal increased oncogenic risk. Individually, these signals may appear non-specific. Together, they form a coherent predictive pattern.

Importantly, cancer risk is not uniform across the body. Different tissues exhibit different vulnerabilities based on exposure, regeneration rate, hormonal influence, and immune access. Predictive science accounts for this heterogeneity by integrating tissue-specific signals rather than relying on universal markers.

"Cancer begins not with a tumor, but with tolerance for instability."

Biomarker Convergence in Cancer Prediction

No single biomarker can predict cancer reliably. Tumor markers detected late reflect established disease rather than emerging risk. Predictive accuracy arises from the convergence of multiple biomarker domains, interpreted dynamically over time.

Molecular and blood-based biomarkers play a central role. Circulating DNA fragments, microRNAs, and protein signatures reveal cellular stress, abnormal turnover, and dysregulated signaling. These markers fluctuate with disease progression, offering insight into trajectory rather than static presence.

Metabolic biomarkers provide additional predictive power. Cancer cells alter energy utilization early, favoring pathways that support rapid growth and survival. Subtle shifts in glucose handling, lipid metabolism, and mitochondrial function may signal early oncogenic processes. These changes often overlap with metabolic disease, underscoring the importance of context-aware interpretation.

Immune biomarkers reveal the state of surveillance and defense. Reduced immune diversity, chronic inflammatory signaling, and altered cytokine balance indicate a weakened ability to eliminate abnormal cells. Predictive models increasingly recognize immune exhaustion as a precursor to malignancy.

Neural and autonomic biomarkers contribute indirectly. Chronic stress alters immune function and metabolic regulation, creating conditions favorable to tumor progression. Predictive frameworks that integrate stress physiology reveal how psychological and biological domains intersect in cancer risk.

Genomic and epigenetic biomarkers refine prediction further. Genetic predisposition modifies susceptibility, while epigenetic drift reflects cumulative exposure and aging. Importantly, epigenetic changes often precede irreversible transformation, making them valuable targets for early intervention.

Eye and vascular biomarkers, though not cancer-specific, reflect systemic health and inflammation. Microvascular changes and altered perfusion patterns often accompany chronic disease states associated with increased cancer risk.

"Cancer prediction emerges not from a single marker, but from the story they tell together."

Artificial Intelligence and Tumor Trajectories

Cancer prediction is a domain where artificial intelligence demonstrates exceptional promise. The sheer complexity of oncogenic processes exceeds human analytical capacity when considered holistically. Machine learning models excel at identifying subtle, high-dimensional patterns across molecular, physiological, and behavioral data.

Predictive systems trained on longitudinal data learn how risk evolves over time. Rather than identifying cancer itself, they estimate **probability of transformation**, **rate of progression**, and **response to intervention**. This shift from detection to forecasting changes the clinical paradigm fundamentally.

Digital twins enable simulation of tumor evolution under different conditions. These models allow researchers and clinicians to explore how inflammation control, metabolic optimization, immune modulation, or targeted therapy influence progression. Such simulation supports proactive rather than reactive care.

Importantly, predictive cancer models must remain explainable. Trust depends on understanding which signals drive risk estimates and how modification may alter outcome. Transparent models empower clinicians and individuals to act confidently.

"Prediction is not about certainty. It is about foresight."

From Early Warning to Oncological Prevention

The ultimate goal of predicting cancer is prevention, not early diagnosis alone. Identifying risk trajectories early allows intervention while cells remain responsive to regulation. Lifestyle modification, immune support, metabolic optimization, and targeted surveillance can reduce transformation probability dramatically.

Predictive insight also personalizes screening. Rather than uniform protocols based on age or population risk, screening intensity and modality can be guided by individual trajectories. This reduces unnecessary procedures while focusing resources where they matter most.

Ethical responsibility is paramount. Cancer prediction carries emotional weight. Risk information must be communicated with care, emphasizing modifiability rather than inevitability. Predictive systems should support informed choice, not anxiety-driven action.

From a public health perspective, predictive oncology reshapes prevention strategies. Population-level risk modeling allows targeted intervention, reducing cancer burden before diagnosis becomes common.

"The greatest cancer intervention may occur before the word 'cancer' is ever spoken."

A New Narrative for Cancer Care

Cancer has long been framed as an enemy to be fought once discovered. Predictive science offers a more nuanced narrative—one of early listening, environmental correction, and systemic support. It teaches us that malignancy is not merely a cellular rebellion, but a failure of communication and regulation.

As predictive tools mature, cancer care will shift upstream. Tumors will no longer define the beginning of care; risk trajectories will. The future of oncology lies not in more aggressive treatment alone, but in earlier understanding and gentler redirection.

Cells whisper before they rebel.

Prediction teaches us to listen early.

"The future of cancer care begins long before the first malignant cell survives."

Chapter 22

Predicting Stroke & Brain Injuries

When the Brain Signals Vulnerability Before the Impact

Stroke and brain injuries are often described as sudden, catastrophic events—moments when life changes irrevocably in an instant. Yet beneath this apparent suddenness lies a long, measurable buildup of vulnerability. Blood vessels stiffen, neural resilience weakens, inflammatory tone rises, and protective reflexes degrade quietly over time. Predictive science reframes stroke and brain injury not as unpredictable accidents, but as **foreseeable outcomes of cumulative imbalance**, detectable well before damage occurs.

The brain depends on uninterrupted blood flow, precise neural coordination, and rapid adaptive capacity. When any of these elements erode, the margin for error narrows. Predictive science seeks to identify this narrowing early, transforming prevention from a reactive response into a proactive safeguard.

"The brain rarely fails without warning.
Its warnings are simply subtle."

The Silent Accumulation of Cerebral Risk

Long before a stroke occurs, the cerebrovascular system undergoes gradual change. Arteries supplying the brain lose elasticity. Microvascular networks become fragile. Endothelial function declines, impairing the brain's ability to regulate blood flow dynamically. These changes often progress without pain or obvious symptoms, allowing risk to accumulate unnoticed.

Predictive science recognizes this silent phase as the most valuable window for intervention. Subtle increases in blood pressure variability, altered cerebral perfusion patterns, and diminished vascular responsiveness signal early risk. These changes may not trigger clinical alarms, yet they steadily reduce the brain's tolerance to stress.

Metabolic dysfunction accelerates this process. Insulin resistance, lipid imbalance, and chronic inflammation compromise vascular integrity and increase clotting tendency. Immune dysregulation further weakens the blood–brain interface, making neural tissue more susceptible to ischemic injury.

Neural signaling patterns also shift during this period. Reduced network adaptability, impaired autonomic regulation, and altered stress response decrease the brain's ability to compensate during sudden physiological challenges. Predictive models reveal that these functional changes often precede structural injury.

Traumatic brain injury risk follows a similar pattern. Reduced reaction time, impaired balance, diminished sensory integration, and cognitive fatigue increase susceptibility to falls, accidents, and impact-related damage. These vulnerabilities often emerge gradually, particularly in aging populations, athletes, and individuals with chronic stress or sleep disruption.

"Stroke and injury are events. Vulnerability is a process."

Biomarker Pathways in Predicting Brain Injury and Stroke

Predicting stroke and brain injury requires integration across multiple biomarker domains. No single signal captures risk fully. Predictive accuracy emerges from **pattern recognition across systems**.

Cardiovascular and hemodynamic biomarkers provide foundational insight. Pulse wave velocity, blood pressure variability, and vascular stiffness reflect cerebrovascular health. Subtle abnormalities in these measures often predict ischemic and hemorrhagic events years in advance.

Heart-signal and ECG biomarkers add predictive depth. Atrial rhythm instability, reduced heart rate variability, and conduction abnormalities increase embolic risk and impair cerebral perfusion. These signals often coexist with silent vascular disease.

Neural and brain-signal biomarkers reveal functional vulnerability. Reduced neural complexity, altered synchronization, and impaired autonomic control indicate diminished capacity to adapt to hypoxia or ischemia. These changes are especially relevant in predicting transient ischemic attacks and recurrent stroke.

Eye and vision-based biomarkers offer a unique window into cerebral microvasculature. Retinal vessel abnormalities mirror cerebral vascular pathology closely. Changes in vessel caliber, branching patterns, and perfusion correlate strongly with stroke risk and cognitive decline.

Metabolic and immune biomarkers further refine prediction. Inflammatory signaling promotes plaque instability and clot formation. Metabolic dysregulation impairs vascular repair mechanisms. Predictive models consistently show that inflammation and metabolic stress often precede cerebrovascular events.

Speech and cognitive biomarkers also contribute indirectly. Subtle changes in articulation, processing speed, or language fluency may reflect early ischemic stress or network inefficiency. These changes are often dismissed as fatigue or aging, yet they hold predictive value when tracked longitudinally.

Genomic and epigenetic factors modify susceptibility and recovery. Genetic predisposition influences coagulation, vascular integrity, and inflammatory response, while epigenetic drift reflects cumulative exposure and aging.

"The brain's future is written in the health of its vessels."

Artificial Intelligence and Risk Trajectory Modeling

The complexity of stroke and brain injury risk makes artificial intelligence indispensable. Machine learning models integrate cardiovascular, neural, metabolic, and behavioral data to estimate risk trajectories rather than isolated probabilities. These models learn how vulnerability accumulates and how it responds to intervention.

Longitudinal monitoring is essential. A single blood pressure reading or imaging study offers limited insight. Predictive systems track trends—gradual stiffening, declining variability, increasing inflammatory tone—that signal rising risk.

Wearable technologies contribute valuable data. Continuous monitoring of heart rhythm, activity, balance, and sleep reveals early decline in protective capacity. When combined with periodic biochemical and imaging data, these signals form a comprehensive risk profile.

Digital twins enable simulation of cerebrovascular futures. Predictive systems can explore how blood pressure control, metabolic optimization, stress reduction, or rehabilitation alters risk trajectory. This simulation transforms prevention into an adaptive, personalized strategy.

Explainability remains critical. Predictive insight must be transparent, allowing clinicians and individuals to understand which factors drive risk and how change can influence outcome. Trust and engagement depend on clarity.

"Prediction becomes powerful when it explains, not merely forecasts."

From Prediction to Neuroprotection

The ultimate goal of predicting stroke and brain injury is **neuroprotection**—preserving brain function before damage occurs. Early identification of risk allows interventions that strengthen vascular health, enhance neural resilience, and restore adaptability.

Lifestyle modification guided by prediction has profound impact. Blood pressure optimization, metabolic control, physical activity, sleep restoration, and stress management all reduce cerebrovascular vulnerability when applied early. Predictive insight ensures these interventions occur before the brain's margin for error is exhausted.

Predictive monitoring also reshapes rehabilitation. Individuals with prior injury can be monitored for secondary risk, guiding personalized recovery strategies and preventing recurrence.

Ethical responsibility is central. Predictive information about brain injury risk must empower rather than alarm. Communication should emphasize modifiability and support informed choice.

From a public health perspective, predictive cerebrovascular monitoring enables proactive resource allocation, targeted prevention programs, and reduced long-term disability burden.

"Protecting the brain begins long before the first insult."

A New Paradigm for Brain Safety

Stroke and brain injury have long been treated as emergencies to be managed after the fact. Predictive science transforms them into **preventable outcomes**, guided by early listening and timely action. By recognizing vulnerability as a process rather than an event, healthcare shifts from reaction to protection.

The brain signals its limits quietly.

Prediction teaches us to listen early and respond wisely.

"The future of brain health depends on how early we act, not how fast we respond."

Chapter 23

Predicting Respiratory & Lung Illnesses

When Breath Begins to Change Long Before It Is Lost

Breathing is the most continuous act of life. It occurs without conscious effort, adapting seamlessly to movement, emotion, environment, and need. Because of this constancy, respiratory decline often goes unnoticed until it becomes disruptive. Predictive science challenges this delay. It reveals that lung and respiratory illnesses rarely emerge suddenly. They unfold gradually, altering airflow, gas exchange, rhythm, and resilience long before breathlessness demands attention.

Respiratory health is inseparable from cardiovascular function, immune balance, metabolic state, neural regulation, and environmental exposure. Predictive science views lung disease not as an isolated failure of airways or alveoli, but as a **systemic trajectory** that can be anticipated, measured, and redirected early.

"The lungs do not fail suddenly. They adapt until adaptation is no longer enough."

The Silent Decline of Respiratory Resilience

Many respiratory illnesses begin with subtle loss of adaptability rather than overt obstruction. Lung tissue becomes less elastic. Airway responsiveness changes. Gas exchange efficiency declines slightly. These changes may not alter resting breathing, but they reduce the system's ability to respond to stress, exertion, or infection.

Predictive science identifies this early decline through patterns rather than symptoms. Slight increases in respiratory rate variability, altered breathing rhythm, reduced oxygen recovery after exertion, and changes in sleep-related breathing patterns signal emerging vulnerability. These changes often precede diagnoses such as asthma, chronic obstructive pulmonary disease, interstitial lung disease, and pulmonary hypertension.

Environmental exposure plays a critical role. Air pollution, occupational hazards, allergens, and smoking create chronic inflammatory stress within lung tissue. Even after exposure ceases, immune and structural changes may persist, gradually reshaping respiratory capacity.

Metabolic dysfunction compounds risk. Insulin resistance, obesity, and systemic inflammation alter respiratory mechanics and immune defense, increasing susceptibility to infection and chronic disease. Sleep disruption further impairs respiratory regulation, reducing nocturnal recovery and amplifying daytime vulnerability.

Infections reveal these hidden weaknesses. Individuals with reduced respiratory resilience experience more severe illness, slower recovery, and higher risk of long-term complications. Predictive science seeks to identify vulnerability **before** infection exposes it.

"Respiratory disease begins with lost reserve, not lost air."

Biomarker Pathways in Respiratory Prediction

Predicting respiratory and lung illness requires integration across physiological, immune, neural, and environmental biomarkers. No single test captures respiratory risk fully. Predictive accuracy emerges from convergence.

Pulmonary function dynamics provide foundational insight. Subtle declines in airflow variability, reduced inspiratory capacity, and delayed recovery after exertion reveal early loss of elasticity and airway control. These changes often precede measurable obstruction.

Oxygenation patterns add further predictive value. Small fluctuations in oxygen saturation during sleep or activity reflect impaired gas exchange and ventilation–perfusion mismatch. These patterns predict progression toward chronic lung disease and sleep-related breathing disorders.

Immune biomarkers play a central role. Chronic low-grade inflammation alters airway responsiveness and tissue repair. Immune imbalance increases susceptibility to infection and accelerates structural damage. Predictive models consistently show that immune dysregulation often precedes chronic respiratory illness.

Neural and autonomic biomarkers further refine prediction. Breathing rhythm is regulated by neural networks sensitive to stress, sleep, and metabolic state. Altered autonomic balance disrupts respiratory control, increasing variability and reducing adaptability.

Cardiovascular biomarkers intersect strongly with respiratory health. Pulmonary circulation depends on vascular integrity and cardiac performance. Heart-signal and pulse biomarkers reveal early pulmonary vascular stress and right-heart strain, often before respiratory symptoms appear.

Speech and voice biomarkers provide indirect yet valuable insight. Changes in breath support, vocal stamina, and speech rhythm reflect respiratory inefficiency. These changes often emerge subtly, particularly in early obstructive and restrictive lung disease.

Eye and microvascular biomarkers reflect systemic oxygenation and inflammatory status. Retinal vessel changes and ocular perfusion patterns correlate with chronic hypoxia and vascular remodeling associated with lung disease.

Genomic and epigenetic factors modify susceptibility. Genetic predisposition influences airway responsiveness and immune regulation, while epigenetic drift reflects cumulative environmental exposure.

"Breathing is controlled by many systems. Prediction listens to all of them."

Artificial Intelligence and Respiratory Trajectories

The dynamic nature of breathing makes respiratory disease particularly suited to AI-driven prediction. Machine learning models analyze continuous respiratory signals, learning patterns that indicate declining resilience rather than overt failure.

Wearable sensors capture breathing rate, rhythm, oxygen saturation, activity tolerance, and sleep-related patterns. When combined with environmental data such as air quality and temperature, predictive systems gain context-aware insight into respiratory stress.

Digital twins enable simulation of respiratory futures. Predictive models can explore how exposure reduction, fitness improvement, immune modulation, or sleep optimization alters long-term lung health. This allows individuals and clinicians to test interventions virtually before applying them in life.

Explainability remains essential. Predictive insight must clarify which factors drive risk and how intervention can restore reserve. Transparency builds trust and supports sustained engagement.

"Prediction matters only when it guides prevention."

From Early Warning to Respiratory Preservation

The ultimate goal of predicting respiratory illness is preservation of breathing capacity and resilience. Early identification of vulnerability allows interventions that strengthen lung function, enhance immune defense, and reduce environmental stress.

Lifestyle and environmental modification guided by prediction has profound impact. Reducing exposure, improving physical conditioning, restoring sleep quality, and managing inflammation preserve respiratory reserve. Predictive insight ensures these actions occur before irreversible remodeling sets in.

Predictive monitoring also reshapes post-infection care. Individuals recovering from severe respiratory illness can be tracked for long-term vulnerability, guiding rehabilitation and preventing chronic decline.

Ethical responsibility remains central. Predictive respiratory data must empower rather than alarm. Breath is deeply tied to emotion and anxiety. Communication must emphasize modifiability and support.

From a public health perspective, predictive respiratory monitoring enables proactive response to pollution, pandemics, and climate-related stress. Healthcare systems can anticipate demand and protect vulnerable populations early.

"To protect breath is to protect life itself."

A New Vision for Lung Health

Respiratory disease has long been treated as a response problem—managing symptoms after decline becomes apparent. Predictive science transforms it into a **resilience problem**, one that can be addressed early through listening, adaptation, and prevention.

Breathing changes quietly before it fails.

Prediction teaches us to hear those changes in time.

"The future of respiratory health lies in preserving reserve, not reacting to loss."

Chapter 24

Predicting Eye-Based Diseases: Glaucoma & Retinopathy

When Vision Begins to Fade Long Before Sight Is Lost

Vision loss is often perceived as a sudden and devastating event. Yet most blinding eye diseases do not steal sight abruptly. They progress quietly, reshaping neural tissue, microvasculature, and cellular metabolism long before the individual becomes aware of any deficit. Predictive science reframes eye-based diseases not as conditions discovered when vision deteriorates, but as **processes that can be anticipated and slowed while sight is still intact.**

Glaucoma and retinopathy exemplify this principle. Both diseases advance silently, damaging neural and vascular structures in the eye while central vision remains deceptively normal. By the time symptoms appear, irreversible injury has often already occurred. Predictive science listens earlier—to subtle changes in ocular structure, function, and systemic interaction—transforming prevention from aspiration into practice.

"Vision is rarely lost suddenly. It withdraws quietly, one signal at a time."

The Silent Pathology of Glaucoma and Retinopathy

Glaucoma is fundamentally a neurodegenerative disease of the optic nerve. While elevated intraocular pressure has long been emphasized, predictive science reveals a broader truth. Glaucoma involves impaired blood flow, mitochondrial dysfunction, altered neural resilience, and susceptibility to mechanical and metabolic stress. Pressure alone does not explain progression, nor does normal pressure guarantee safety.

Retinopathy, particularly diabetic retinopathy, reflects microvascular failure. Capillaries weaken, leak, and close. Neural tissue becomes hypoxic. Inflammation disrupts repair. These changes develop gradually, often without affecting visual acuity until late stages. Predictive science recognizes that retinopathy is not merely a complication of diabetes, but a **systemic vascular and metabolic signal** visible through the eye.

Both conditions share a defining feature: long asymptomatic phases. During this time, the eye compensates. Alternative pathways preserve central vision. Neural plasticity masks damage. This compensation creates the illusion of health while vulnerability deepens.

Predictive science identifies this phase as the critical window for intervention. Subtle thinning of retinal nerve fiber layers, altered perfusion patterns, microvascular irregularities, and changes in ocular metabolism all precede functional loss. These changes are measurable with modern imaging and signal analysis, long before conventional screening detects disease.

"The eye compensates beautifully—until it can no longer do so."

Biomarker Pathways in Ocular Disease Prediction

Predicting glaucoma and retinopathy requires integration across ocular, neural, vascular, and systemic biomarkers. The eye does not exist in isolation. It reflects the health of the brain, heart, metabolism, and immune system.

Structural ocular biomarkers provide foundational insight. Gradual thinning of retinal nerve fiber layers and ganglion cell complexes signals early neurodegeneration in glaucoma. In retinopathy, microaneurysms, capillary dropout, and subtle edema reflect early vascular compromise. These changes often precede visual field loss by years.

Functional visual biomarkers add predictive depth. Altered contrast sensitivity, delayed visual processing, and impaired adaptation to light reflect early neural dysfunction. Eye movement patterns and fixation stability reveal subtle deficits in neural control and visual integration.

Vascular biomarkers are central to both diseases. Reduced ocular perfusion pressure, altered vessel caliber, and impaired autoregulation reflect systemic vascular dysfunction. These changes correlate strongly with cardiovascular and cerebrovascular risk, reinforcing the eye's role as a window into systemic health.

Metabolic and immune biomarkers further refine prediction. Chronic hyperglycemia, insulin resistance, and inflammation damage retinal vessels and neural tissue. Predictive models show that inflammatory burden and metabolic variability often precede overt retinopathy.

Neural biomarkers connect ocular disease to broader neurodegeneration. The retina shares embryological origin with the brain. Changes in retinal neural layers often mirror changes in cortical and subcortical structures. Predictive frameworks increasingly treat glaucoma as part of a wider neurodegenerative spectrum rather than an isolated eye disease.

Genomic and epigenetic factors modify vulnerability. Genetic predisposition influences optic nerve resilience and vascular integrity, while epigenetic drift reflects cumulative exposure to stress, aging, and metabolic imbalance.

"The eye reveals what the rest of the body struggles to hide."

Artificial Intelligence and Predictive Ophthalmology

The complexity and subtlety of ocular changes make artificial intelligence indispensable in predictive ophthalmology. High-resolution retinal imaging generates vast amounts of data beyond human interpretation. AI systems excel at identifying micro-patterns that signal early disease trajectory.

Machine learning models trained on retinal images can predict glaucoma progression, retinopathy risk, and even systemic diseases such as cardiovascular and neurological disorders. These models identify patterns invisible to clinicians, transforming routine eye exams into predictive health assessments.

Longitudinal analysis is particularly powerful. Tracking subtle changes over time reveals progression patterns that static images cannot capture. Predictive systems learn individual baselines, detecting deviation rather than relying on population thresholds.

Digital twins of ocular systems enable simulation of disease progression under different conditions. Predictive models can explore how pressure control, metabolic optimization, vascular support, or neuroprotective strategies influence long-term visual outcome.

Explainability remains essential. Predictive insights must be interpretable to guide clinical decision-making and patient understanding. Transparent models build trust and enable early, targeted intervention.

"Prediction turns observation into foresight."

From Early Detection to Vision Preservation

The ultimate goal of predicting glaucoma and retinopathy is not earlier diagnosis alone, but **long-term preservation of vision**. When vulnerability is identified early, interventions are often simpler and more effective. Pressure modulation, metabolic control, vascular support, and lifestyle modification slow progression dramatically when applied before extensive damage occurs.

Predictive monitoring empowers individuals. Awareness of risk allows proactive engagement, adherence to preventive strategies, and informed planning. Importantly, prediction does not imply inevitability. Many individuals with elevated risk may never experience significant vision loss if protective measures are implemented early.

Ethical responsibility is central. Vision loss carries emotional weight. Predictive information must be communicated with care, emphasizing modifiability and support rather than fear. Autonomy and informed choice must guide predictive care.

From a public health perspective, predictive ophthalmology offers scalable prevention. Eye screening is non-invasive, widely accessible, and cost-effective. Integrating predictive analytics into routine eye care could prevent millions of cases of avoidable blindness worldwide.

"Protecting vision begins long before sight is threatened."

A New Paradigm for Eye Health

Glaucoma and retinopathy teach a powerful lesson about disease: the most damaging processes are often the quietest. Predictive science gives voice to these quiet changes, allowing intervention while vision remains intact.

The eye does not wait for disease to announce itself.It signals imbalance patiently.

Prediction teaches us to listen early and protect sight for a lifetime.

"The future of vision lies not in restoring what is lost, but in preserving what remains."

Chapter 25

Predicting Mental Health Disorders

When the Mind Signals Distress Long Before Crisis Emerges

Mental health disorders are often recognized only when suffering becomes visible—when mood collapses, behavior changes abruptly, or functioning deteriorates. Yet psychological distress rarely appears without warning. Long before diagnosis, the mind and body signal imbalance through subtle shifts in emotion regulation, cognition, sleep, physiology, and behavior. Predictive science reframes mental health not as a sudden breakdown, but as a **gradual divergence from psychological resilience**, one that can be observed, measured, and addressed early.

The mind does not exist in isolation. Mental health emerges from continuous interaction between neural circuits, hormonal systems, immune balance, metabolism, social context, and lived experience. Predictive science listens across these domains, revealing early vulnerability long before crisis demands intervention.

"Mental illness rarely begins with collapse. It begins with quiet misalignment."

The Gradual Drift from Psychological Resilience

Psychological resilience is the capacity to adapt to stress, regulate emotion, maintain cognitive clarity, and recover from adversity. When this capacity erodes, distress accumulates quietly. Sleep becomes fragmented. Emotional responses grow less flexible. Attention narrows. Motivation fluctuates. These changes are often dismissed as stress or fatigue, yet they represent early warning signals of deeper imbalance.

Predictive science recognizes that disorders such as depression, anxiety, bipolar disorder, schizophrenia, post-traumatic stress disorder, and attention-related conditions do not emerge suddenly. They evolve through identifiable phases of vulnerability. During these phases, individuals may function outwardly while internal regulation becomes increasingly strained.

Neural signaling patterns shift subtly. Emotional regulation circuits lose coordination. Reward pathways respond less robustly. Stress-response systems become hyperactive or blunted. Over time, these changes reduce the mind's ability to adapt, increasing the likelihood of symptomatic breakdown.

Environmental and social factors amplify this drift. Chronic stress, trauma, isolation, sleep deprivation, and sustained uncertainty alter neural plasticity and hormonal balance. Predictive science integrates these contextual influences rather than treating mental illness as purely internal dysfunction.

"The mind adapts until adaptation itself becomes exhausting."

Biomarker Pathways in Mental Health Prediction

Predicting mental health disorders requires a holistic approach to biomarkers that reflect both brain function and systemic regulation. No single signal captures psychological risk fully. Predictive accuracy emerges from convergence across neural, physiological, behavioral, and contextual domains.

Neural and brain-signal biomarkers provide foundational insight. Altered connectivity in emotional and cognitive networks, reduced signal variability, and disrupted oscillatory patterns reflect early dysregulation. These changes often precede mood symptoms and cognitive impairment.

Speech and language biomarkers offer a uniquely accessible window into mental state. Subtle changes in speech rhythm, pitch variability, word choice, and pause patterns reflect emotional tone, cognitive load, and psychomotor activity. These changes often appear early in depression, anxiety, bipolar disorder, and psychosis, even when individuals consciously mask distress.

Sleep biomarkers are among the strongest predictors of mental health trajectories. Disrupted circadian rhythms, fragmented sleep, and altered sleep architecture precede mood disorders and exacerbate vulnerability. Predictive models consistently show that sleep disruption often comes before emotional collapse rather than resulting from it.

Autonomic and cardiovascular biomarkers add another layer. Reduced heart rate variability reflects impaired stress regulation. Persistent sympathetic activation signals chronic psychological strain. These physiological changes often precede clinical anxiety and depressive disorders.

Metabolic and immune biomarkers further refine prediction. Inflammatory signaling alters neurotransmission and mood regulation. Metabolic imbalance affects energy availability and cognitive clarity. Predictive frameworks increasingly recognize inflammation and metabolic stress as contributors to mental illness rather than secondary effects.

Behavioral biomarkers complete the picture. Changes in activity patterns, social engagement, digital behavior, and response to routine tasks reveal early withdrawal, impulsivity, or cognitive fatigue. These signals are often more reliable than self-report, particularly in early stages.

Genomic and epigenetic factors modify susceptibility and recovery. Genetic predisposition influences neurotransmitter regulation and stress response, while epigenetic changes reflect trauma, chronic stress, and environmental exposure.

"The mind speaks through many signals.
Prediction listens to all of them."

Artificial Intelligence and Psychological Trajectories

The complexity and individuality of mental health make artificial intelligence particularly valuable for prediction. Machine learning models integrate diverse data streams, learning how psychological vulnerability evolves over time. Rather than labeling disorders, predictive systems estimate **risk trajectories**, identifying periods of increased vulnerability and resilience.

Longitudinal monitoring is central to this approach. A single assessment cannot capture mental health accurately. Predictive systems track change—gradual shifts in sleep, speech, behavior, and physiology that accumulate meaning. These models learn individual baselines, reducing false alarms and enhancing relevance.

Digital twins offer a powerful future tool. Predictive models can simulate how lifestyle changes, therapy, medication, or environmental modification influence mental health trajectories. This allows proactive planning and personalized intervention rather than trial-and-error care.

Explainability remains essential. Mental health prediction must be transparent, compassionate, and interpretable. Individuals and clinicians must understand why risk is changing and how action can influence outcome. Prediction without understanding risks harm.

"Prediction must support dignity, not replace judgment."

From Early Insight to Psychological Well-Being

The ultimate goal of predicting mental health disorders is not early diagnosis alone, but **preservation of psychological well-being**. Early identification of vulnerability allows intervention when adaptation is still possible. Counseling, lifestyle adjustment, social support, sleep restoration, and stress management are most effective when applied early.

Predictive monitoring also reduces stigma. When mental health is framed as a dynamic process rather than a sudden failure, individuals are more likely to seek support. Prediction normalizes vulnerability and emphasizes care over crisis.

Ethical responsibility is paramount. Mental health data is deeply personal. Predictive systems must prioritize consent, privacy, and autonomy. Risk information should empower choice, not define identity.

From a societal perspective, predictive mental health care transforms public health. Early support reduces crisis-driven care, hospitalization, and long-term disability. Communities become proactive rather than reactive.

"Mental health is not the absence of distress,
but the ability to recover."

A New Vision for Mental Health Care

Mental health disorders have long been treated after suffering becomes visible. Predictive science offers a new vision—one of early listening, compassionate response, and sustained resilience. It teaches us that the mind signals imbalance patiently, waiting to be understood.

The future of mental health care lies not in reacting to breakdown, but in protecting balance.

The mind does not break suddenly.

It asks for support quietly. Prediction teaches us to hear that request in time.

"The future of mental health depends on how early we choose to care."

SECTION IV

Technologies Transforming Health

Chapter 26

Wearable & Implantable Biosensing Systems

When the Body Becomes a Continuous Source of Predictive Intelligence

Healthcare has traditionally relied on snapshots—brief clinical encounters, isolated measurements, and episodic testing. Between these moments, the body lives, adapts, struggles, and compensates in silence. Wearable and implantable biosensing systems transform this paradigm. They allow the body to be observed continuously, revealing physiological narratives that were previously invisible. Predictive science thrives on such continuity. It requires not isolated numbers, but patterns unfolding over time.

Wearable and implantable sensors represent a fundamental shift in how health is understood. They convert biology into dynamic signals, translating internal states into streams of data that can be analyzed, interpreted, and acted upon long before disease becomes visible.

"The body is always speaking. Sensors give it a language we can hear."

From Episodic Monitoring to Continuous Physiology

Traditional diagnostics capture health at rest, often under artificial conditions. Blood tests, imaging, and clinical examinations reveal valuable information, but they miss the dynamic nature of living systems. Predictive science requires a different lens—one that observes how the body responds to stress, recovery, sleep, movement, emotion, and environment.

Wearable biosensors provide this lens. By continuously tracking physiological signals such as heart rhythm, movement, respiration, temperature, and oxygenation, they reveal fluctuations that reflect resilience or vulnerability. These fluctuations matter more than static values. A heart that adapts well to stress signals health. A system that becomes rigid or erratic signals risk.

Implantable biosensors extend this capability deeper into the body. They measure signals inaccessible to external devices, such as intracardiac activity, neural firing patterns, biochemical concentrations, and localized tissue responses. These systems operate silently, often unnoticed by the individual, yet they provide unparalleled insight into internal regulation.

Predictive science values continuity because disease rarely emerges abruptly. Physiological drift occurs gradually. Continuous sensing captures this drift early, allowing intervention while adaptation is still possible.

"Health is not a state. It is a pattern."

Biosensing Modalities and Predictive Insight

Wearable and implantable systems capture a wide spectrum of biological signals, each contributing to predictive understanding. Cardiovascular sensors reveal rhythm stability, variability, and hemodynamic response. Respiratory sensors capture breathing patterns, recovery efficiency, and stress response. Motion sensors reveal activity patterns, balance, and fatigue. Thermal sensors detect inflammatory processes and metabolic shifts.

More advanced systems integrate biochemical sensing. Continuous glucose monitoring has already transformed diabetes care, but predictive science extends this approach to other molecules. Emerging sensors track lactate, cortisol, electrolytes, and inflammatory markers, revealing metabolic and stress dynamics in real time.

Neural sensing systems represent one of the most powerful frontiers. Implantable and wearable neural interfaces capture brain and peripheral nerve activity, revealing changes in cognition, emotion, motor control, and autonomic regulation. These signals hold immense predictive value for neurological, psychiatric, and neurodegenerative disorders.

Importantly, predictive power does not come from any single signal. It emerges from **signal interaction**. A mild change in heart rate may be meaningless alone, but when paired with altered sleep, reduced activity, and increased stress markers, it becomes significant. Biosensing systems enable this integrative view.

"Prediction lives in relationships between signals, not in signals themselves."

Artificial Intelligence as the Interpreter of Biosignals

The volume and complexity of biosensing data exceed human analytical capacity. Artificial intelligence acts as the interpreter, transforming raw signals into meaningful insight. Machine learning models identify patterns, trends, and deviations that predict disease risk, progression, or recovery.

These models learn individual baselines. Rather than comparing a person to population averages, predictive systems track how an individual changes over time. This personalization dramatically improves accuracy and relevance. What matters is not whether a value is normal, but whether it is changing in a concerning direction.

Digital twins emerge naturally from this integration. Continuous biosensing feeds personalized computational models that simulate physiological behavior. These twins allow exploration of "what-if" scenarios—how sleep improvement, exercise, medication, or stress reduction alters future health trajectories.

Explainability remains essential. Predictive insights must be interpretable, not opaque. Individuals and clinicians need to understand why risk is changing and how action can influence outcome. Trust in biosensing systems depends on transparency and reliability.

"Data without meaning is noise. Intelligence gives it purpose."

Ethical, Human, and Societal Dimensions

Wearable and implantable biosensing systems raise profound ethical questions. Continuous monitoring touches privacy, autonomy, consent, and psychological well-being. Predictive science must ensure that sensing empowers individuals rather than surveils them.

Data ownership is central. Individuals must retain control over their biological data. Predictive systems should operate as partners, not overseers. Consent must be ongoing and informed, particularly for implantable devices that operate invisibly.

Psychological impact also matters. Continuous health data can provoke anxiety if poorly contextualized. Predictive insight must be framed as guidance, not judgment. Systems should emphasize trends and modifiability rather than fixed labels.

Equity remains a critical concern. Predictive biosensing must not become a privilege limited to affluent populations. Scalable, affordable sensing technologies are essential to ensure that predictive healthcare benefits all communities, including rural and low-resource settings.

From a societal perspective, biosensing systems reshape healthcare delivery. Hospitals become monitoring hubs rather than primary diagnostic sites. Care shifts upstream, focusing on prevention rather than crisis response. Public health strategies evolve from reactive to anticipatory.

"Technology must serve humanity, not redefine it."

Toward a Living, Predictive Healthcare System

Wearable and implantable biosensing systems transform healthcare into a living process—one that adapts continuously, learns from experience, and responds early. They align naturally with the philosophy of predictive science, which seeks to understand health as a dynamic journey rather than a binary state.

As biosensing technology matures, the boundary between body and system dissolves. The body becomes a continuous source of insight, guiding care in real time. Disease no longer arrives unannounced. It signals its approach patiently, waiting to be heard.

Predictive science gives us the tools to listen.

"The future of healthcare will not be scheduled. It will be continuous."

Chapter 27

Nature-Inspired Optimization Algorithms

When Intelligence Learns from Life Itself

Long before artificial intelligence existed, nature solved problems of extraordinary complexity. Survival demanded efficiency, adaptability, resilience, and foresight. Over millions of years, biological systems learned how to optimize energy use, navigate uncertainty, recover from disruption, and evolve under pressure. Predictive science recognizes that these strategies are not merely biological curiosities; they are computational blueprints.

Nature-inspired optimization algorithms emerge from this realization. They do not attempt to overpower complexity through brute force. Instead, they emulate the principles through which natural systems explore possibilities, adapt to constraints, and converge toward optimal solutions. In healthcare, where biological systems themselves are the subject of prediction, these algorithms form a natural bridge between computation and life.

"Nature does not compute faster. It computes wiser."

Why Nature Solves What Equations Cannot

Traditional optimization methods assume stable landscapes, clear gradients, and well-defined objectives. Biological systems violate these assumptions constantly. The human body operates in noisy, uncertain environments where objectives change and trade-offs are unavoidable. Predictive science therefore requires algorithms that tolerate ambiguity, adapt dynamically, and seek balance rather than absolute perfection.

Nature-inspired algorithms excel under these conditions. They explore multiple solutions simultaneously, avoid premature convergence, and continuously balance exploration with exploitation. Rather than committing early to a single path, they remain flexible, adjusting strategy as new information emerges.

In predictive healthcare, this flexibility is essential. Disease prediction involves conflicting objectives—accuracy versus interpretability, sensitivity versus specificity, early warning versus false alarms. Nature-inspired optimization models these trade-offs naturally, evolving toward solutions that satisfy multiple criteria rather than optimizing a single metric.

These algorithms also reflect biological reality. The same principles that govern immune response, neural learning, and evolutionary adaptation guide computational search. This alignment makes them particularly well-suited for modeling living systems.

"Life optimizes for survival, not perfection."

Evolution, Swarms, and Collective Intelligence

Many nature-inspired algorithms draw from evolutionary principles. Genetic algorithms simulate variation, selection, and inheritance. Candidate solutions evolve over generations, adapting to constraints and improving fitness. This mirrors biological evolution, where diversity ensures resilience and adaptability.

Swarm intelligence offers another powerful metaphor. Ant colonies, bird flocks, fish schools, and bee hives demonstrate how simple agents following local rules can produce globally optimal behavior. In healthcare prediction, swarm-based algorithms excel at feature selection, parameter tuning, and pattern discovery in complex datasets.

These systems do not rely on centralized control. Instead, intelligence emerges from interaction. This property aligns closely with biological systems, where regulation is distributed rather than hierarchical. Predictive science benefits from this decentralization, particularly when modeling multi-organ interactions and systemic disease.

Neural inspiration extends beyond artificial neural networks. Brain-inspired optimization emphasizes adaptability, memory, and learning from sparse feedback. These principles guide algorithms that adjust continuously as new patient data arrives, supporting real-time predictive refinement.

"Intelligence emerges where interaction replaces control."

Optimization in Predictive Healthcare Systems

Nature-inspired optimization plays a central role across predictive healthcare pipelines. Feature selection is one of its most impactful applications. Biomedical datasets often contain thousands of variables, many redundant or irrelevant. Nature-inspired algorithms identify optimal feature subsets that preserve predictive power while enhancing interpretability.

Model optimization represents another critical application. Predictive models must balance complexity and generalization. Overly complex models risk overfitting, while overly simple ones miss subtle patterns. Nature-inspired algorithms navigate this balance dynamically, adapting model structure to data behavior.

In disease prediction, these algorithms optimize not just accuracy but **clinical relevance**. They can be designed to prioritize early detection, minimize false reassurance, or emphasize robustness across populations. This multi-objective optimization aligns naturally with healthcare priorities.

Nature-inspired methods also support personalization. Each individual represents a unique optimization landscape. Algorithms that adapt to individual baselines and trajectories outperform static population-based models. This personalization is central to predictive medicine's promise.

"The best model is not the most complex one, but the one that adapts."

Futuristic Integration with Digital Twins and AI

As predictive science advances, nature-inspired optimization becomes integral to digital twin systems. Digital twins simulate physiological processes, disease progression, and intervention outcomes. Optimization algorithms continuously adjust these simulations, ensuring alignment with real-world data.

In the future, predictive systems will evolve autonomously. As biosensing data streams in, optimization algorithms will refine models in real time, learning from outcomes and updating predictions continuously. This creates a self-improving healthcare intelligence system.

Hybrid approaches are emerging, combining deep learning with nature-inspired optimization. While deep learning excels at representation, optimization algorithms guide training, feature weighting, and decision boundaries. Together, they form robust, adaptive predictive systems.

Importantly, these algorithms support **explainable optimization**. Unlike opaque black-box tuning, nature-inspired methods reveal evolutionary pathways and trade-offs, supporting transparency and trust.

"The future of AI is not domination, but cooperation—with nature as teacher."

Ethics, Responsibility, and Biological Respect

Drawing inspiration from nature carries responsibility. Nature-inspired algorithms must respect the complexity of living systems rather than reduce them to abstract problems. Optimization should support health, not enforce rigid definitions of normality.

Ethical design ensures that optimization objectives reflect human values. Predictive healthcare must prioritize well-being, dignity, and equity. Nature-inspired algorithms, with their emphasis on balance and adaptability, offer a philosophical alignment with these goals.

There is also humility in learning from nature. These algorithms remind us that intelligence did not begin with machines. It evolved through life itself.

"When we learn from nature, we learn restraint as well as power."

A Biological Intelligence for Predictive Science

Nature-inspired optimization algorithms represent more than computational tools. They embody a philosophy of problem-solving rooted in adaptation, resilience, and balance. In predictive science, they enable systems that listen, learn, and evolve—just as living organisms do.

By aligning computation with biology, predictive healthcare becomes not just technologically advanced, but biologically informed. This alignment is essential for building systems that truly understand health.

Nature has been optimizing life for billions of years.

Predictive science is only beginning to listen.

"The most advanced intelligence may be the one that remembers where it came from."

Chapter 28

Synthetic Data & Digital Patients

When Healthcare Learns Before Real Lives Are Touched

Modern medicine stands at a paradox. It needs vast amounts of data to predict disease accurately, yet it must protect privacy, dignity, and safety. Real patient data is scarce, fragmented, biased, and ethically constrained. Predictive science resolves this tension through a powerful idea: creating data that behaves like life without being life itself.

Synthetic data and digital patients represent a foundational shift in healthcare intelligence. They allow systems to learn, test, and evolve before decisions affect real human beings. Instead of waiting for disease to occur, predictive science simulates its possibilities. Instead of experimenting on populations, it experiments on models. In doing so, it accelerates discovery while preserving trust.

"The safest place to learn about disease is before it touches a human life."

Why Real Data Alone Is Not Enough

Traditional healthcare analytics depend heavily on real patient data. While invaluable, this data carries inherent limitations. It reflects historical bias, incomplete observation, inconsistent measurement, and unequal access to care. Rare diseases remain underrepresented. Early disease stages are poorly captured. Longitudinal continuity is often missing.

Predictive science demands something different. It requires data that spans full disease trajectories, including stages that rarely reach clinics. It requires balanced representation across populations, environments, and biological variability. It requires the ability to explore futures that have not yet occurred.

Synthetic data fulfills these needs. Generated through statistical modeling, machine learning, and biological simulation, synthetic data preserves the structure, relationships, and dynamics of real data without exposing individual identities. It enables safe experimentation at scale.

Importantly, synthetic data is not random. When designed correctly, it reflects biological plausibility, clinical realism, and temporal coherence. Predictive models trained on such data learn patterns of disease evolution rather than memorizing historical accidents.

"Synthetic data does not replace reality. It prepares us for it."

Digital Patients as Living Models

Digital patients extend synthetic data from static records into dynamic entities. A digital patient is a computational representation of a human being, capable of simulating physiology, disease progression, and response to intervention over time. These models integrate biomarkers, signals, behaviors, genetics, and environment into coherent systems.

Unlike traditional simulations, digital patients are not fixed. They evolve. As new data arrives, their internal states update. As interventions are applied, their trajectories change. This adaptability makes them ideal tools for predictive science.

Digital patients enable exploration of "what-if" scenarios. What if intervention occurs earlier? What if lifestyle changes are sustained? What if treatment is delayed or altered? These questions can be explored safely and repeatedly without risk.

In predictive healthcare, digital patients act as intermediaries between data and decision. They absorb uncertainty, explore alternatives, and present probabilistic futures rather than deterministic outcomes.

"Digital patients allow medicine to think before it acts."

Synthetic Data in Disease Prediction and AI Training

Artificial intelligence thrives on diversity and volume. Synthetic data provides both. By generating millions of realistic patient trajectories, predictive models learn rare patterns, early signals, and complex interactions that real datasets cannot supply alone.

In disease prediction, synthetic data fills critical gaps. Early-stage Parkinson's disease, preclinical cancer, silent metabolic dysfunction, and subclinical mental health disorders are often absent from real datasets. Synthetic augmentation reconstructs these stages, enabling earlier prediction.

Feature interaction becomes clearer through synthetic exploration. Models can test how biomarkers interact under controlled variation, revealing causal relationships rather than correlations alone. This improves robustness and interpretability.

Synthetic data also supports fairness. Bias present in real datasets can be identified and corrected during generation. Populations historically underrepresented in research can be modeled explicitly, improving equity in predictive systems.

Importantly, validation remains essential. Synthetic data must be continuously anchored to real-world evidence. Predictive science treats synthetic and real data as complementary, not competing sources of truth.

"The value of synthetic data lies not in imitation, but in illumination."

Ethical Power and Responsibility

Synthetic data and digital patients carry profound ethical advantages. They reduce dependence on invasive testing, protect privacy, and minimize harm during research and development. Predictive models can be stress-tested extensively before deployment.

Yet responsibility remains. Synthetic systems must not drift into biological fantasy. Models must be grounded in empirical evidence and continuously audited. Transparency in generation methods is essential to maintain trust.

Digital patients also challenge traditional consent models. While no real individual is represented, decisions derived from these models affect real lives. Predictive science must ensure that simulated outcomes are communicated with humility and uncertainty acknowledged openly.

The ethical promise of synthetic systems lies in their ability to **protect while preparing**. They allow medicine to learn without exploiting vulnerability.

"Ethical intelligence learns without causing harm."

The Future: A World of Simulated Health

In the coming decades, synthetic data and digital patients will become foundational to healthcare. Before a new treatment is approved, it will be tested across millions of digital lives. Before public health policy is enacted, its impact will be simulated across populations. Before personalized care plans are prescribed, their outcomes will be explored in silico.

Hospitals will maintain libraries of digital patients representing their communities. Clinicians will consult simulations alongside clinical judgment. Researchers will discover patterns not by waiting for decades of outcomes, but by modeling them responsibly.

Most importantly, individuals will benefit. Care will become anticipatory rather than reactive. Interventions will be tailored not only to who a person is, but to who they are likely to become.

Synthetic data does not remove humanity from medicine.

It gives humanity more time to act wisely.

"The future of healthcare may be simulated—but its impact will be profoundly real."

Chapter 29

Federated Learning & Edge AI in Healthcare

When Intelligence Travels to the Data Instead of Taking Data Away

For decades, healthcare intelligence followed a centralizing logic. Data was collected, transferred, stored, and analyzed in distant servers. This approach delivered breakthroughs, yet it also introduced new risks—privacy erosion, latency, inequity, and dependence on infrastructure unavailable to much of the world. Predictive science demands a different architecture, one aligned with trust, speed, and local relevance.

Federated learning and edge AI embody this shift. They reverse the flow of intelligence. Instead of extracting sensitive health data from individuals and institutions, intelligence moves to where the data lives. Learning becomes distributed, privacy-preserving, and continuous. In this model, prediction does not wait for data to travel. It happens at the source of life itself.

"The future of intelligence is not centralized. It is shared."

The Limits of Centralized Intelligence

Centralized AI systems require massive data aggregation. In healthcare, this poses significant challenges. Patient data is sensitive, regulated, and often siloed. Transferring it introduces legal complexity, security risk, and ethical tension. Moreover, centralized models struggle to reflect local variation in population health, environment, and care practices.

Predictive science recognizes that health is contextual. Disease manifests differently across geographies, cultures, and lifestyles. Centralized models trained on limited or biased datasets risk producing predictions that generalize poorly. The result is intelligence that is powerful yet disconnected from lived reality.

Latency further limits centralized systems. Predictive insight loses value when delayed. In critical care, wearable monitoring, and rural health settings, waiting for cloud-based analysis can be impractical or unsafe. Predictive science requires immediacy.

Federated learning and edge AI emerge as natural solutions to these limitations. They preserve privacy, respect locality, and enable real-time intelligence without sacrificing learning capacity.

"Healthcare intelligence must be close enough to care."

Federated Learning: Collective Intelligence Without Data Exchange

Federated learning enables multiple institutions, devices, or communities to train shared models without exchanging raw data. Each participant trains a local model on its own data. Only model updates—not sensitive records—are shared and aggregated. Knowledge travels, not data.

In healthcare, this paradigm is transformative. Hospitals, clinics, and devices collaborate without violating privacy. Rare disease patterns can be learned across institutions without exposing individual identities. Predictive models become richer while remaining ethically grounded.

Federated learning also enhances robustness. Models trained across diverse environments learn generalizable patterns rather than institution-specific artifacts. This diversity strengthens prediction and reduces bias.

Crucially, federated systems support continuous learning. As new data arrives locally, models adapt incrementally. Predictive systems evolve alongside populations rather than becoming obsolete.

Yet federated learning is not merely a technical solution. It represents a philosophical shift toward **collective intelligence built on trust**.

"Federation turns isolation into collaboration."

Edge AI: Intelligence at the Point of Life

Edge AI brings computation directly to devices—wearables, implantables, medical equipment, and local clinics. Instead of streaming raw data to the cloud, devices analyze signals locally, generating predictive insight in real time.

In predictive healthcare, this proximity matters. Continuous biosensing produces vast data streams. Edge AI filters, interprets, and responds immediately. It detects anomalies, trends, and early warning signals without delay.

Edge intelligence is especially powerful in resource-limited settings. Rural clinics, mobile health units, and home-based care often lack reliable connectivity. Edge AI enables predictive monitoring without dependence on constant network access, democratizing advanced care.

Edge systems also enhance resilience. They continue functioning during outages, disasters, or infrastructure disruption. Predictive science thus becomes more robust, less fragile, and more human-centered.

Importantly, edge AI aligns with personalization. Models adapt to individual baselines locally, learning what is normal for one person rather than relying on population averages.

"When intelligence lives at the edge, care becomes immediate."

Federated Edge Intelligence in Predictive Science

The convergence of federated learning and edge AI creates a powerful architecture for predictive healthcare. Edge devices perform local prediction and learning. Federated systems coordinate collective improvement. Together, they form a living network of intelligence.

Wearable biosensors detect early physiological drift. Edge AI interprets signals instantly. Federated learning aggregates insights across populations, refining prediction without exposing individuals. This architecture supports early detection, continuous adaptation, and ethical integrity.

Digital twins benefit significantly from this approach. Edge data keeps twins synchronized with real physiology. Federated updates ensure that twin models reflect collective learning while remaining personalized.

This architecture also supports rapid response to emerging threats. During outbreaks or environmental crises, predictive models update across networks without centralized bottlenecks. Healthcare intelligence becomes agile rather than reactive.

"Distributed intelligence mirrors distributed life."

Ethics, Trust, and Governance

Federated and edge systems embed ethics into architecture. Privacy is preserved by design rather than policy alone. Data sovereignty is respected. Individuals retain control over their biological information.

Yet governance remains essential. Model updates must be validated. Bias must be monitored. Accountability must be clear. Predictive science requires transparent protocols for participation, aggregation, and oversight.

Trust is the currency of predictive healthcare. Federated and edge systems earn trust by minimizing intrusion and maximizing benefit.

When individuals see that intelligence serves them without extracting from them, engagement deepens.

Equity is also enhanced. By reducing dependence on centralized infrastructure, federated edge systems bring predictive care to underserved communities. Intelligence becomes portable, scalable, and inclusive.

"Ethical systems are those that protect by design."

Toward a Decentralized Future of Health Intelligence

The future of healthcare intelligence will not be built in distant data centers alone. It will live in homes, on bodies, within communities. Federated learning and edge AI make this future possible.

Prediction becomes continuous yet discreet. Learning becomes collective yet private. Care becomes anticipatory yet personal.

This architecture aligns perfectly with predictive science's core promise—to understand health as it unfolds, not after it fails.

The intelligence of the future will not demand our data.

It will earn our trust.

"The most powerful healthcare intelligence is the one people allow to exist."

Chapter 30

Blockchain & Intelligent Health Records

When Trust Becomes the Foundation of Predictive Healthcare

Healthcare has always struggled with memory. Patient histories are fragmented across hospitals, clinics, devices, and lifetimes. Records are incomplete, inconsistent, and often inaccessible when they matter most. Predictive science, which depends on continuity and integrity of information, cannot thrive on fractured memory. It requires a system that remembers accurately, securely, and ethically—across time, institutions, and technologies.

Blockchain and intelligent health records answer this need. They do not merely digitize healthcare data; they redefine how trust, ownership, and continuity are embedded into healthcare intelligence. In predictive medicine, where decisions are made before disease manifests, **trust in data becomes as important as data itself.**

"Prediction is only as reliable as the truth it remembers."

The Fragility of Conventional Health Records

Traditional electronic health records were designed primarily for documentation and billing, not for prediction. They capture events, not trajectories. They record diagnoses, not preclinical signals. Worse, they exist in silos. A patient's health narrative is scattered across institutions, often irretrievable during critical moments.

This fragmentation undermines predictive science. Without longitudinal continuity, early patterns remain invisible. Without data integrity, predictive models lose reliability. Without patient control, trust erodes.

Moreover, centralized record systems create single points of failure. Data breaches, manipulation, unauthorized access, and institutional dependency threaten both privacy and accuracy. Predictive healthcare cannot rest on fragile infrastructure.

Blockchain technology offers a fundamentally different architecture—one that treats health data not as institutional property, but as **a verifiable, patient-centered timeline of truth**.

"Healthcare fails when memory fails."

Blockchain as a Trust Infrastructure

Blockchain introduces a decentralized ledger where records are immutable, time-stamped, and verifiable. Once information is recorded, it cannot be altered without consensus. This immutability is critical for predictive science, where historical integrity directly affects future inference.

In intelligent health records, blockchain does not store raw medical data directly. Instead, it anchors data references, permissions, and audit trails. Actual health data may reside securely off-chain, while blockchain ensures that access, modification, and provenance are transparent and tamper-proof.

This architecture restores trust. Patients can verify who accessed their data and why. Clinicians can trust the authenticity of records. Predictive models can rely on data lineage, knowing that what they learn from has not been silently altered.

Blockchain also enables interoperability. Different healthcare providers can contribute to a shared patient record without surrendering control to a central authority. Predictive science benefits from this continuity, gaining access to complete longitudinal narratives rather than fragmented episodes.

"When data cannot be trusted, prediction becomes speculation."

Intelligent Health Records: From Storage to Understanding

Intelligent health records go beyond static documentation. They integrate analytics, predictive models, and contextual understanding directly into the record itself. Instead of merely storing information, these systems **interpret it continuously**.

In predictive healthcare, intelligent records act as living entities. They update as new biosensor data arrives, as laboratory values fluctuate, and as behavioral patterns evolve. Predictive algorithms analyze trends within the record, flagging early risk signals and generating foresight rather than alerts after failure.

Blockchain enhances this intelligence by ensuring that insights are derived from trusted data. Predictive recommendations are traceable to validated inputs. This traceability is essential for clinical confidence and ethical accountability.

Importantly, intelligent records shift ownership back to individuals. Patients become stewards of their health narratives. They grant and revoke access dynamically, participate in predictive decisions, and understand how their data shapes their future care.

"A health record should not just remember the past. It should protect the future."

Blockchain, AI, and Predictive Integrity

As artificial intelligence becomes deeply integrated into healthcare decision-making, the integrity of data pipelines becomes critical. Predictive models trained on compromised or biased data can cause harm silently and at scale.

Blockchain introduces accountability into AI systems. Model training data, updates, and decision logic can be audited. This transparency supports explainability and regulatory oversight, especially in high-stakes predictive applications.

Federated learning systems benefit from blockchain coordination. Model updates exchanged across institutions can be verified, tracked, and governed transparently. This ensures that collective intelligence evolves responsibly.

Smart contracts further enhance predictive healthcare. Automated rules can govern data sharing, consent, and intervention thresholds. For example, predictive alerts may trigger only when predefined ethical and clinical criteria are met, reducing unnecessary alarm and preserving autonomy.

"Ethical AI requires ethical memory."

Privacy, Autonomy, and Human Dignity

Blockchain-based health records embed privacy not as an afterthought, but as a structural principle. Data access is permissioned, time-bound, and revocable. Individuals retain sovereignty over their biological information.

This autonomy is essential in predictive science. Predictive insights can influence identity, behavior, and opportunity. Individuals must control how and when such insights are generated and shared.

Intelligent records must also communicate uncertainty. Prediction is probabilistic, not deterministic. Blockchain-backed transparency ensures that risk estimates are contextualized, traceable, and open to challenge.

From a societal perspective, blockchain-enabled health records support equity. They reduce dependence on institutional power, enable cross-border continuity of care, and protect vulnerable populations from data exploitation.

"Dignity in healthcare begins with control over one's own story."

Toward a Trusted Predictive Healthcare Ecosystem

The future of healthcare intelligence depends not only on advanced algorithms, but on **trustworthy foundations**. Blockchain and intelligent health records provide these foundations. They ensure that predictive systems learn from accurate memory, respect autonomy, and operate transparently.

In such a system, prediction becomes a shared endeavor. Patients, clinicians, and systems collaborate around a trusted narrative of health. Decisions are informed by continuity rather than snapshots, foresight rather than hindsight.

When memory is protected, prediction becomes meaningful. When trust is embedded, intelligence becomes humane.

"The future of predictive healthcare will be written on chains of trust."

Chapter 31

Robotics & Predictive Surgery

When Surgery Thinks Before the Scalpel Touches the Body

Surgery has long been defined by precision of the human hand and the judgment of the surgeon's mind. Yet even the most skilled surgeon operates within limits—limited visibility, limited time, limited ability to foresee how tissues will respond, heal, or fail. Predictive science expands these limits. Robotics and predictive surgery transform surgical care from a reactive intervention into a **foreseen, simulated, and continuously optimized process**.

In predictive surgery, the operation does not begin in the operating room. It begins weeks, months, or even years earlier—inside data, models, and simulations that anticipate risk, personalize strategy, and guide decision-making before a single incision is made.

"The best surgery is the one that already understands the body before it enters it."

From Mechanical Assistance to Cognitive Surgical Systems

Early surgical robots were tools—extensions of human motion designed to enhance precision and stability. Predictive surgery moves far beyond this role. Robotics becomes cognitive, informed by patient-specific data, predictive models, and real-time feedback.

Predictive surgical systems integrate imaging, biosignals, genomic profiles, and physiological trends into a unified preoperative intelligence. Before surgery, the system simulates multiple procedural pathways, anticipating bleeding risk, tissue response, healing potential, and complication likelihood. These simulations inform not only how surgery is performed, but whether it is needed at all.

Robotics enables execution of these optimized strategies with consistency and control. Tremor elimination, micron-level precision, and adaptive motion allow surgeons to operate with enhanced confidence. Predictive models guide robotic systems in adjusting force, trajectory, and timing based on tissue feedback rather than rigid preprogramming.

Importantly, robotics does not replace the surgeon. It augments human decision-making, reducing cognitive and physical burden while preserving clinical judgment.

"Robotics extends the surgeon's reach; prediction extends the surgeon's foresight."

Patient-Specific Prediction Before the First Cut

Predictive surgery centers on personalization. No two bodies heal the same way. Predictive models analyze patient-specific risk factors such as metabolic status, vascular health, immune balance, tissue quality, and genetic predisposition to estimate surgical outcomes.

Digital twins play a crucial role here. A patient's digital twin simulates the planned procedure repeatedly under varying conditions. Surgeons can explore alternative approaches, assess risk trade-offs, and select strategies that minimize trauma and maximize recovery.

This foresight changes surgical decision-making fundamentally. Some surgeries may be postponed, modified, or avoided entirely when predictive models suggest poor benefit-to-risk ratios. Others may be optimized through prehabilitation—improving metabolic health, reducing inflammation, or strengthening tissue resilience before intervention.

Predictive insights also improve informed consent. Patients understand not only what will be done, but what is likely to happen afterward. Surgery becomes a shared, data-informed decision rather than a leap into uncertainty.

"Prediction transforms consent from hope into understanding."

Intraoperative Intelligence and Real-Time Adaptation

During surgery, predictive systems continue to operate. Robotic platforms integrate real-time sensor data—force feedback, tissue resistance, bleeding patterns, and physiological response—into adaptive control loops. AI models predict tissue behavior milliseconds ahead, allowing micro-adjustments that reduce injury.

This real-time prediction is especially powerful in complex procedures involving delicate structures such as nerves, vessels, and organs. Robotics guided by predictive intelligence can recognize subtle deviations from expected tissue response, alerting surgeons before damage occurs.

Augmented visualization enhances this process. Predictive overlays highlight risk zones, optimal pathways, and dynamic changes in anatomy. Surgeons operate not just on what they see, but on what the system anticipates.

Predictive surgery also reduces variability. Outcomes become less dependent on fatigue, stress, or environmental factors. Consistency improves safety and equity across surgical care.

"In predictive surgery, the body teaches the system while the system protects the body."

Postoperative Prediction and Recovery Optimization

The impact of predictive surgery extends beyond the operating room. Postoperative recovery is itself a predictive process. Continuous monitoring through wearables and biosensors tracks healing, inflammation, mobility, and physiological stress.

Predictive models anticipate complications before symptoms appear. Early warning of infection, thrombosis, or delayed healing enables timely intervention, reducing morbidity and length of stay. Rehabilitation plans adapt dynamically based on recovery trajectory rather than fixed timelines.

Robotics also supports recovery. Assistive robotic devices guide rehabilitation exercises, adjust intensity based on fatigue and healing, and prevent overexertion. Predictive insights ensure that recovery is progressive, safe, and personalized.

"Healing is not a phase. It is a forecast."

Ethics, Responsibility, and Surgical Trust

Predictive surgery raises profound ethical questions. Decisions influenced by algorithms must remain accountable to human values. Surgeons retain responsibility for judgment, interpretation, and compassion.

Transparency is essential. Predictive models must explain why certain strategies are recommended. Uncertainty must be communicated honestly. Robotics should enhance trust, not obscure it.

Equity remains a critical concern. Predictive surgical technologies must not widen healthcare disparities. Accessibility, training, and cost must be addressed deliberately to ensure that advanced care benefits all populations.

"The most advanced surgery is still a human act."

Toward a Predictive Surgical Future

The future of surgery lies not in sharper tools alone, but in **earlier understanding**. Robotics and predictive science together redefine surgery as an intelligent, anticipatory process—one that respects the body's complexity and prepares for its response.

In this future, surgery is safer, recovery is smoother, and uncertainty is reduced. The scalpel is guided not only by the hand, but by insight.

The operation begins long before the incision.

The healing begins before the wound exists.

"When surgery learns to predict, the body learns to heal better."

Chapter 32

IOT Hospitals & Smart Clinics

When Care Becomes an Intelligent, Living Environment

Hospitals have traditionally been places of reaction. Patients arrive when symptoms worsen, clinicians respond to crises, and technology supports intervention after decline becomes visible. Predictive science reimagines this environment entirely. In an IoT-enabled hospital or smart clinic, care does not wait for alarms or emergencies. It listens continuously, learns silently, and acts early.

The Internet of Things transforms healthcare spaces into intelligent ecosystems. Devices, sensors, systems, and people communicate seamlessly, creating an environment that understands health as it unfolds. Predictive science thrives in such environments because they generate the continuity, context, and connectivity required to anticipate disease rather than merely respond to it.

"The hospital of the future does not wait for illness. It notices imbalance."

From Static Infrastructure to Living Systems

Conventional hospitals operate through compartmentalization. Departments function independently. Data flows slowly. Equipment is monitored episodically. Predictive science requires a different architecture—one where the hospital itself becomes a sensing, thinking organism.

IoT hospitals integrate sensors across beds, rooms, corridors, devices, and wearables. Vital signs, movement patterns, environmental conditions, equipment performance, and staff workflows are observed continuously. These signals do not exist in isolation. They are fused into contextual understanding.

A patient's physiological signals are interpreted alongside room temperature, noise levels, light exposure, medication timing, and staff interaction. Predictive models learn how these factors interact, identifying subtle contributors to recovery or decline. Care becomes adaptive rather than protocol-driven.

Smart clinics extend this philosophy beyond large hospitals. Community clinics, diagnostic centers, and home-care hubs connect seamlessly into the healthcare network. Predictive insight follows the patient rather than remaining confined to institutional walls.

"Intelligence emerges when systems stop working alone."

Predictive Care in Real Time

IoT environments enable real-time prediction. Continuous data streams allow models to detect early deviation from healthy trajectories. A slight increase in heart rate variability, reduced mobility, altered sleep patterns, or environmental stress may signal emerging risk long before clinical deterioration.

Predictive alerts in smart hospitals are not alarms in the traditional sense. They are anticipatory insights delivered to clinicians in context. Rather than reacting to crisis, care teams adjust intervention proactively—modifying treatment, environment, or support.

Resource optimization is another critical benefit. Predictive models anticipate patient flow, staffing needs, equipment utilization, and supply demand. Hospitals become efficient without becoming impersonal. Predictive insight reduces burnout by aligning workload with real-time need.

In infection control, IoT systems monitor movement, air quality, surface usage, and hygiene compliance. Predictive models identify risk patterns early, preventing outbreaks rather than managing them after spread occurs.

"Prediction turns hospitals from responders into protectors."

Integration with Wearables, Edge AI, and Digital Twins

IoT hospitals do not operate in isolation. They integrate seamlessly with wearable biosensors, edge AI systems, and digital patients. Data flows bi-directionally. What is learned in the hospital informs home care, and what is observed at home informs clinical decision-making.

Edge AI enables local processing, reducing latency and preserving privacy. Predictive insight is generated close to the patient, while federated systems ensure collective learning across institutions. Digital twins update continuously, reflecting real-world physiology and environmental influence.

Smart clinics leverage these tools to extend predictive care into underserved regions. Remote monitoring reduces unnecessary admissions. Early intervention prevents escalation. Predictive science thus reshapes access, not just technology.

"Care follows the patient, not the building."

Human-Centered Intelligence and Clinical Trust

Technology alone does not create a smart hospital. Trust does. Predictive systems must enhance human care, not replace it. Clinicians remain central decision-makers, supported by insight rather than overwhelmed by data.

User-centered design is essential. Predictive insights are delivered clearly, with explanation and uncertainty acknowledged. Systems prioritize relevance over volume, ensuring that intelligence supports rather than distracts.

Patients also become participants. Smart environments inform individuals about their own recovery, empowering engagement and adherence. Transparency builds confidence and reduces anxiety.

Ethical governance underpins these systems. Data privacy, consent, and fairness must be embedded into design. Predictive care must respect dignity and autonomy at every step.

"A smart hospital is one that listens—to data and to people."

Toward an Intelligent Care Continuum

IoT hospitals and smart clinics represent more than technological advancement. They signal a philosophical shift from episodic care to continuous stewardship of health. Predictive science transforms healthcare spaces into environments that anticipate, adapt, and protect.

In this future, hospitals are no longer places one visits only when ill. They are nodes in a living network of care, supporting health across time and context.

The walls become transparent. The care becomes continuous. The intelligence becomes humane.

"The hospital of the future will be less about machines and more about understanding."

SECTION V

Humanity, Ethics & Policy

Chapter 33

Ethics of Predictive Healthcare

When Knowing the Future Demands Moral Wisdom

Predictive healthcare marks one of the most profound shifts in the history of medicine. For the first time, healthcare systems are not merely reacting to disease but anticipating it—sometimes years before symptoms emerge. This power to foresee carries extraordinary promise, but it also carries responsibility. Knowing the future of health is not ethically neutral. It reshapes identity, decision-making, freedom, and trust.

Ethics in predictive healthcare is not an accessory added after technological development. It is the foundation upon which predictive science must stand. Without ethical grounding, prediction risks becoming surveillance, optimization risks becoming coercion, and foresight risks becoming fear.

"The power to predict is also the power to influence—and influence demands responsibility."

Prediction, Autonomy, and the Right Not to Know

At the heart of predictive ethics lies autonomy. Predictive systems may reveal risk long before individuals feel ill. While this knowledge can empower, it can also burden. Not every person wishes to know their future health risks, especially when uncertainty remains.

Ethical predictive healthcare respects the right to choose—not only what to know, but when and how to know it. Consent must be dynamic rather than one-time. Individuals should retain the freedom to pause, limit, or withdraw from predictive insight without penalty.

Prediction must never become destiny. Risk estimates are probabilistic, not deterministic. Ethical systems communicate uncertainty clearly, avoiding language that transforms possibility into inevitability. Individuals must be supported in understanding that prediction informs choice; it does not replace it.

The right not to know is as important as the right to know. Predictive healthcare must protect both equally.

"Freedom in healthcare includes the freedom to remain unburdened by foresight."

Privacy, Surveillance, and Human Dignity

Predictive healthcare thrives on data—continuous, intimate, deeply personal data. Biosignals, behaviors, speech, movement, and even emotional patterns become inputs for prediction. Without ethical restraint, this depth of observation risks crossing into surveillance.

Ethical predictive systems embed privacy by design. Data collection must be proportional, purposeful, and transparent. Individuals must understand what is collected, why it is collected, and how it is used. Ownership of health data must remain with the individual, not the system.

Predictive monitoring must never become constant judgment. Health data reflects vulnerability, not value. Systems must be designed to support care, not enforce conformity. The goal of prediction is protection, not control.

Human dignity demands that predictive healthcare sees people as partners, not subjects. Intelligence must serve humanity, not observe it from above.

"When prediction forgets dignity, it ceases to be healthcare."

Bias, Fairness, and Social Responsibility

Predictive systems learn from data shaped by history, inequality, and access. Without ethical vigilance, these systems risk amplifying existing biases—misrepresenting risk, excluding marginalized populations, and reinforcing inequity.

Ethical predictive healthcare requires continuous bias auditing, diverse data representation, and inclusive design. Prediction must work for all populations, not only those historically visible in healthcare datasets.

Fairness also extends to access. Predictive healthcare must not become a privilege reserved for the technologically connected or economically advantaged. Ethical design prioritizes scalability, affordability, and deployment in low-resource settings.

From a societal perspective, predictive healthcare reshapes responsibility. When disease becomes predictable, responsibility shifts from individual blame to collective care. Ethical systems emphasize support, prevention, and shared accountability rather than moral judgment.

"Equity is not optional when intelligence guides care."

Psychological Impact and the Ethics of Foreknowledge

Knowing future health risk changes how people live. It can motivate positive change, but it can also create anxiety, hypervigilance, or identity reduction. Ethical predictive healthcare must address this psychological dimension openly.

Predictive insights should be framed as guidance, not verdicts. Support systems—clinical, psychological, and social—must accompany prediction. Information without support can harm more than it helps.

Language matters. How risk is communicated shapes perception. Ethical systems avoid catastrophic framing and emphasize modifiability, resilience, and agency. The goal is empowerment, not fear.

Prediction should open doors to care, not close doors to opportunity. Ethical safeguards must prevent discrimination in employment, insurance, and social participation based on predictive health data.

"Foreknowledge without compassion becomes burden."

Accountability, Transparency, and Trust

As predictive systems influence clinical decisions, accountability becomes essential. Who is responsible when prediction fails? Who explains when outcomes diverge from forecasts? Ethical healthcare requires clear lines of responsibility.

Transparency builds trust. Predictive models must be explainable, auditable, and open to challenge. Clinicians must understand how predictions are generated. Patients must understand why recommendations are made.

Ethical governance ensures that predictive systems evolve responsibly. Oversight committees, regulatory frameworks, and public engagement are necessary to guide development and deployment.

Trust is fragile. Once lost, it is difficult to regain. Ethical design prioritizes trust not as a feature, but as a principle.

"Trust is the most important biomarker of predictive healthcare."

A Moral Compass for the Future of Medicine

Predictive healthcare offers unprecedented opportunity to reduce suffering, extend healthy life, and preserve dignity. Yet its success depends not on algorithms alone, but on moral wisdom.

Ethics ensures that prediction remains a gift rather than a burden. It reminds us that health is not merely a system to be optimized, but a human experience to be respected.

As predictive science advances, ethics must advance with it—not behind it.

The future of healthcare will know more than ever before. Its greatness will be measured by how wisely it uses that knowledge.

"The highest form of intelligence is care guided by conscience."

Chapter 34

Regulations & Responsible AI in Medicine

When Intelligence Must Be Governed to Truly Heal

As artificial intelligence moves from laboratories into clinics, homes, and bodies, it reshapes not only how medicine is practiced, but how responsibility is defined. Predictive healthcare systems increasingly influence diagnosis, prevention, treatment planning, and even life decisions. This influence demands governance that is as intelligent as the systems it seeks to guide.

Regulation in predictive medicine is not about slowing innovation. It is about ensuring that innovation remains aligned with human values, clinical safety, and social trust. Responsible AI is the bridge between technological possibility and ethical legitimacy.

"In medicine, power without governance is risk."

Why Medicine Demands a Higher Standard of AI Responsibility

Healthcare differs fundamentally from other AI application domains. Errors do not merely inconvenience users; they affect bodies, identities, and lives. Predictive systems may act before symptoms appear, influencing decisions under uncertainty. This amplifies both their potential benefit and their potential harm.

Traditional medical regulation evolved around drugs, devices, and procedures. Predictive AI introduces a new category—systems that learn, adapt, and evolve. Unlike static tools, these systems change over time, creating challenges for certification, validation, and accountability.

Responsible AI in medicine therefore requires a shift from **one-time approval to continuous oversight**. Safety is not a moment; it is a process. Predictive models must be monitored for drift, bias, and unintended consequences throughout their lifecycle.

Importantly, responsibility does not rest solely with developers. Clinicians, institutions, regulators, and society share stewardship of predictive systems. Governance must reflect this shared responsibility.

"A system that learns continuously must be governed continuously."

Principles of Responsible Predictive AI

Responsible AI in medicine rests on foundational principles that guide design, deployment, and use. Transparency ensures that predictive insights can be understood and questioned. Explainability allows clinicians and patients to see why a recommendation exists, not merely what it suggests.

Accountability ensures that decisions influenced by AI remain traceable to human oversight. Predictive systems must support, not replace, clinical judgment. When outcomes diverge from predictions, responsibility must be clear and reviewable.

Fairness addresses bias and representation. Predictive models trained on incomplete or skewed data risk amplifying inequity. Responsible regulation demands rigorous evaluation across populations, continuous bias assessment, and corrective mechanisms.

Safety and robustness protect against failure under real-world conditions. Predictive systems must perform reliably across environments, populations, and time. Rare but high-impact errors must be anticipated and mitigated.

Privacy and data protection preserve dignity. Predictive healthcare relies on deeply personal data. Regulation must ensure that data is collected minimally, used purposefully, and protected rigorously.

"Responsible AI is not defined by capability, but by restraint."

Regulatory Evolution in the Age of Prediction

Global regulatory frameworks are evolving to meet the challenges of AI-driven medicine. Traditional device classifications struggle to accommodate adaptive algorithms. Predictive systems may change behavior as they learn, challenging static approval models.

Emerging regulatory approaches emphasize **risk-based classification**. Systems that influence high-stakes decisions face stricter scrutiny than those offering low-risk guidance. This proportionality enables innovation while protecting patients.

Regulators increasingly recognize the importance of post-deployment monitoring. Real-world performance data informs ongoing assessment, enabling early detection of bias, drift, or unintended harm. Regulation becomes a dialogue rather than a gate.

International harmonization is critical. Predictive healthcare systems often cross borders digitally. Fragmented regulation risks inconsistency, confusion, and inequity. Collaborative frameworks support shared standards while respecting local context.

Importantly, regulation must remain adaptive. Overly rigid rules risk freezing innovation. Overly permissive frameworks risk erosion of trust. Responsible regulation balances flexibility with protection.

"Good regulation evolves with technology, not behind it."

Clinical Responsibility and Human Oversight

No predictive system should operate without human oversight. Clinicians remain accountable for decisions, even when supported by AI. Responsible AI augments expertise rather than replacing it.

Training becomes essential. Clinicians must understand predictive systems well enough to interpret, question, and contextualize their output. Regulation must therefore extend beyond technology to education and professional standards.

Predictive recommendations must be presented as guidance, not commands. Interfaces should encourage reflection, not compliance. Responsible design supports shared decision-making between clinician and patient.

When AI systems err, mechanisms for reporting, review, and correction must exist. Learning from failure is as important as celebrating success.

"In medicine, responsibility cannot be automated."

Societal Trust and the Future of Predictive Governance

Public trust is the cornerstone of predictive healthcare. Without trust, individuals will resist participation, limiting data quality and system effectiveness. Regulation plays a central role in building and maintaining this trust.

Transparency with the public matters. People must understand how predictive systems work, what they do, and what they do not do. Fear thrives in opacity; trust grows in clarity.

Responsible AI also demands public engagement. Societal values should inform governance. Predictive healthcare affects everyone, and its rules should reflect collective priorities.

Ultimately, regulation is not an obstacle to innovation—it is its enabler. Systems that are trusted are adopted. Systems that are accountable endure.

"The future of predictive medicine depends not on intelligence alone, but on legitimacy."

Toward a Responsible Predictive Future

Predictive science has the power to transform healthcare profoundly. Whether it does so wisely depends on how responsibly it is governed. Regulation and responsible AI ensure that prediction remains aligned with care, dignity, and justice.

In this future, intelligence advances hand in hand with ethics. Innovation proceeds with humility. And healthcare becomes not only smarter, but safer and more humane.

Prediction may reveal what lies ahead.

Responsibility determines whether that future heals.

"The measure of progress is not how far intelligence can go, but how carefully it is guided."

Chapter 35

Predictive Science For Rural & Low-Resource Communities

When the Future of Healthcare Must Reach Everyone

Healthcare inequality is one of the most persistent challenges of the modern world. While cities advance rapidly toward personalized, technology-driven care, rural and low-resource communities often remain dependent on delayed diagnosis, limited access, and crisis-driven intervention. Predictive science carries a profound responsibility in this context. Its true success will not be measured by sophistication alone, but by **reach, equity, and impact where care is most scarce.**

Predictive science has the potential to reverse long-standing healthcare disparities. By anticipating disease early, reducing dependence on infrastructure-heavy interventions, and enabling decentralized care, it offers rural communities something traditional medicine often cannot: time, foresight, and agency.

"A healthcare future that does not include rural lives is not a future—it is a failure."

The Structural Reality of Rural Healthcare

Rural and low-resource communities face a distinct constellation of challenges. Geographic isolation delays access to care. Shortage of specialists limits diagnostic capability. Infrastructure constraints restrict laboratory testing, imaging, and continuous monitoring. Economic pressures reduce preventive engagement, forcing individuals to seek care only when symptoms become severe.

These conditions create a reactive healthcare cycle. Diseases are detected late. Complications are common. Treatment is expensive and disruptive. Predictive science disrupts this cycle by shifting focus upstream—toward early signals that can be detected with minimal resources.

Importantly, rural communities often possess strengths overlooked by centralized healthcare models. Strong social networks, continuity of lifestyle patterns, and deep local knowledge provide valuable context for prediction. Predictive science must learn from these realities rather than impose urban assumptions.

'Prediction works best when it respects the environment in which life unfolds."

Low-Cost Signals, High-Value Insight

Predictive healthcare for low-resource settings does not require expensive machines or complex laboratories. Many of the most powerful predictive signals are already present in daily life. Pulse patterns, speech changes, movement, sleep, breathing rhythm, and behavioral consistency carry rich information about health trajectories.

Simple sensors, basic smartphones, and community health workers can collect meaningful data. Edge AI enables local interpretation without reliance on constant connectivity. Predictive models can operate offline, updating when connectivity becomes available.

Wearable biosensors designed for affordability and durability allow continuous monitoring without hospital dependence. Community clinics equipped with predictive tools become early warning hubs rather than crisis centers.

Crucially, predictive science reduces the need for repeated travel to distant facilities. Care comes to the community rather than the community chasing care.

"In low-resource settings, intelligence must be light, local, and reliable."

Community-Centered Predictive Models

Predictive science must adapt to local context to succeed. Models trained exclusively on urban or hospital-based data risk misinterpretation in rural environments. Responsible predictive systems incorporate local data, cultural patterns, diet, climate, occupation, and lifestyle.

Federated learning plays a critical role here. Communities contribute to collective intelligence without surrendering data ownership. Local patterns inform global models, while global insights refine local prediction.

Community health workers become key partners in predictive care. Equipped with predictive tools, they identify early risk, guide preventive action, and coordinate referral when needed. This integration elevates local capacity rather than replacing it.

Traditional knowledge also deserves respect. Practices such as pulse observation, symptom narratives, and experiential assessment align naturally with predictive philosophy. Modern predictive science does not erase these traditions; it amplifies them with validation and foresight.

"The most sustainable healthcare is the one that grows within the community."

Disease Prediction Where Burden Is Highest

Rural and low-resource communities often carry disproportionate disease burden. Cardiovascular disease, diabetes, respiratory illness, maternal complications, infectious disease sequelae, and mental health conditions frequently go undetected until advanced stages.

Predictive science enables early identification of vulnerability. Subtle metabolic drift predicts diabetes. Pulse variability signals cardiovascular risk. Breathing patterns indicate respiratory decline. Behavioral changes reveal mental health stress. Predictive monitoring allows intervention before disease becomes disabling.

Maternal and child health benefit particularly from prediction. Early detection of anemia, preeclampsia risk, fetal distress, and developmental delay saves lives where emergency care is distant.

Predictive systems also support outbreak anticipation. Changes in respiratory patterns, fever trends, and community movement signal emerging infectious threats. Early response prevents spread and reduces mortality.

"In places where care arrives late, prediction must arrive early."

Ethics, Trust, and Cultural Sensitivity

Deploying predictive science in vulnerable communities requires deep ethical sensitivity. Technology must empower, not exploit. Data must serve the community, not extract from it. Consent must be informed, contextual, and continuous.

Trust is built through transparency and participation. Communities must understand what predictive systems do, what they do not do, and how insights are used. Predictive care should be framed as support, not surveillance.

Language matters. Risk communication must be culturally appropriate and empowering. Prediction should inspire prevention, not fear. Community leaders, health workers, and families must be engaged as co-stewards of predictive care.

"Healthcare succeeds when communities trust it as their own."

A Vision of Equitable Predictive Care

Predictive science offers an unprecedented opportunity to democratize healthcare. It reduces dependence on expensive infrastructure, centralizes intelligence without centralizing control, and prioritizes prevention where it matters most.

In a predictive future, rural clinics become intelligent nodes of care. Community health workers become agents of foresight. Individuals gain understanding of their own health trajectories. Disease burden shifts from crisis to prevention.

This vision is not utopian. It is achievable—if predictive science chooses inclusion as a core principle rather than an afterthought.

The true measure of predictive healthcare will not be how advanced it becomes in cities, but how deeply it improves life in the most remote places.

"A healthcare revolution is only complete when it reaches the last mile."

Chapter 36

The Global Economics of Preventive Healthcare

When the Cost of Care Is Replaced by the Value of Health

Modern healthcare systems around the world share a common paradox. They spend unprecedented amounts of money, yet struggle to keep populations healthy. Budgets expand, technologies advance, and treatments improve, but disease burden continues to rise. The reason lies not in lack of effort, but in misplaced timing. Most healthcare expenditure occurs after disease has already taken hold. Predictive science offers a different economic logic—one where investment moves upstream, and value is created by preventing loss rather than repairing damage.

Preventive healthcare is not merely a clinical philosophy; it is an economic transformation. It reshapes how societies allocate resources, how governments plan policy, and how individuals experience the cost of living well.

"The most expensive healthcare system is the one that waits."

The Hidden Cost of Reactive Medicine

Reactive healthcare carries costs far beyond hospital bills. Chronic disease reduces productivity, increases disability, and strains families. Late diagnosis leads to complex treatment pathways, prolonged hospital stays, and long-term dependency on care systems. These indirect costs often exceed direct medical expenditure.

Global health data consistently shows that a small fraction of the population with advanced chronic disease consumes a disproportionate share of healthcare resources. Cardiovascular disease, diabetes, cancer, respiratory illness, and neurodegenerative disorders dominate spending precisely because they are detected late and managed over long periods.

Predictive science exposes the inefficiency of this model. When disease trajectories are visible early, the cost curve changes dramatically. Early intervention is almost always less expensive than late-stage treatment. Prevention reduces not only medical cost, but economic disruption at every level of society.

"Healthcare becomes unaffordable when disease becomes inevitable."

Prediction as an Economic Multiplier

Preventive healthcare powered by predictive science acts as an economic multiplier. Small investments in early detection, monitoring, and lifestyle support generate disproportionately large savings over time. These savings compound across populations and generations.

Predictive systems reduce emergency admissions, shorten hospital stays, and decrease the need for high-cost interventions. They enable targeted screening rather than blanket testing, optimizing resource allocation. Healthcare shifts from volume-driven activity to outcome-driven value.

The workforce benefits directly. Healthy populations are productive populations. Reduced disease burden translates into fewer sick days, longer working lives, and sustained cognitive and physical capacity. Predictive healthcare thus becomes a driver of economic resilience rather than a financial drain.

Insurance models also transform. Risk becomes manageable rather than catastrophic. Predictive insights allow insurers to support prevention instead of pricing for failure. When aligned ethically, this reduces premiums, stabilizes systems, and expands coverage.

"Prevention is not a cost. It is an investment with compounding returns."

National Economies and Predictive Policy

At the national level, predictive healthcare reshapes public finance. Governments currently allocate large portions of budgets to managing chronic disease. Predictive science enables a gradual shift from treatment-heavy expenditure to prevention-focused policy.

Predictive public health surveillance anticipates disease trends, enabling early response. Infrastructure investment becomes strategic rather than reactive. Resources are directed where future burden is greatest, not where crisis has already occurred.

Low- and middle-income countries stand to gain significantly. These nations often face a dual burden of infectious disease sequelae and rising chronic illness. Predictive science allows them to leapfrog costly reactive systems, adopting decentralized, prevention-first models that are economically sustainable.

Importantly, predictive healthcare supports fiscal stability. Reduced healthcare volatility enables better long-term planning. Economic shocks caused by epidemics, disability surges, and workforce decline become more manageable.

"A healthy population is the strongest economic policy."

Industry, Innovation, and New Economic Models

Predictive healthcare also transforms the healthcare industry itself. Value shifts from episodic treatment to continuous health management. New economic models emerge around monitoring, prevention, and optimization rather than procedures alone.

Technology companies, healthcare providers, and policymakers must align incentives carefully. Preventive systems succeed when they reward outcomes, not activity. Predictive care requires reimbursement models that recognize avoided disease as value created.

Pharmaceutical economics also evolve. Drugs increasingly target early disease stages or risk modification. Companion diagnostics and predictive markers guide precise use, reducing waste and improving outcomes.

Digital health platforms, biosensing technologies, and AI services become core infrastructure rather than optional add-ons. Their economic value lies not in novelty, but in sustained reduction of disease burden.

"The future healthcare economy rewards what does not happen."

Equity, Sustainability, and Global Responsibility

Economic transformation without equity risks deepening inequality. Predictive healthcare must be designed to reduce, not widen, global health gaps. Preventive tools must be affordable, scalable, and accessible across income levels.

From a sustainability perspective, preventive healthcare reduces environmental strain. Fewer hospitalizations, reduced pharmaceutical waste, and optimized resource use lower healthcare's ecological footprint. Healthy societies consume fewer emergency resources and adapt better to climate-related stress.

Global collaboration amplifies these benefits. Shared predictive insights, ethical data governance, and cooperative policy enable collective resilience. Disease does not respect borders; neither should prevention.

"The economics of prevention is the economics of shared survival."

Redefining Value in Healthcare

At its core, the economics of preventive healthcare challenges a fundamental assumption: that healthcare is a cost center. Predictive science reframes it as a value generator—creating time, productivity, stability, and dignity.

When health is preserved, families remain intact, communities remain functional, and societies remain adaptive. The true return on preventive investment is not only measured in currency, but in continuity of life.

Healthcare systems that learn to predict will spend less repairing damage and more sustaining potential.

The future economy will not be built on treating illness alone. It will be built on protecting health before it is lost.

"The wealthiest societies of the future will be those that learned to prevent."

SECTION VI

Beyond The Present: The Future of Human Health

Chapter 37

Longevity Science & Reversing Biological Aging

When Aging Becomes a Predictable, Modifiable Process

For most of human history, aging has been accepted as an unavoidable decline—an irreversible march toward fragility, disease, and dependence. Medicine has largely treated aging as a backdrop rather than a target, intervening only when age-related diseases emerge. Predictive science challenges this narrative fundamentally. It reveals aging not as a fixed destiny, but as a **biological process with measurable signals, variable trajectories, and modifiable pace**.

Longevity science does not seek immortality. It seeks vitality. Its goal is not merely to extend lifespan, but to preserve function, resilience, and dignity across time. Predictive science provides the lens through which aging becomes understandable, forecastable, and, increasingly, reversible in its early stages.

"Aging is not a cliff. It is a slope—and slopes can be reshaped."

Chronological Age vs Biological Time

Chronological age counts years. Biological age measures wear. Predictive science exposes the profound difference between the two. Two individuals of the same chronological age may differ biologically by decades. One may exhibit cellular resilience, metabolic flexibility, and cognitive clarity, while the other shows inflammation, organ decline, and frailty.

Biological aging manifests through measurable signals long before disease appears. Cellular repair slows. Mitochondrial efficiency declines. Immune surveillance weakens. Vascular elasticity decreases. Neural adaptability narrows. These changes accumulate quietly, often dismissed as "normal aging" when they are, in fact, **early indicators of accelerated decline.**

Predictive science identifies these signals early. Epigenetic drift, telomere dynamics, proteomic imbalance, metabolic inflexibility, and autonomic rigidity all contribute to biological aging trajectories. When monitored longitudinally, they reveal whether an individual is aging slowly, rapidly, or reversibly.

Crucially, biological age is dynamic. It responds to sleep, nutrition, movement, stress, environment, and meaning. Predictive insight transforms aging from a passive experience into an active, informed process.

"We do not age because time passes. We age because systems stop adapting."

The Biology of Aging as a Predictive System

Aging is not caused by a single mechanism. It emerges from interacting systems gradually losing coordination. Predictive science approaches aging as a network problem rather than an isolated failure.

Cellular aging begins with accumulated damage and reduced repair capacity. DNA repair becomes less efficient. Protein quality control weakens. Cellular senescence increases, releasing inflammatory signals that affect neighboring tissue. Predictive models detect these shifts long before tissue failure becomes apparent.

Metabolic aging follows. Cells lose flexibility in energy utilization. Insulin sensitivity declines. Mitochondrial output becomes inconsistent.

These changes increase vulnerability to chronic disease but also signal early aging acceleration.

Immune aging, or immunosenescence, reduces the body's ability to respond to threats and remove damaged cells. Chronic low-grade inflammation emerges, often described as inflammaging. Predictive science tracks immune balance to forecast disease susceptibility and recovery potential.

Neural aging manifests as reduced plasticity, slower processing, and diminished stress resilience. These changes often precede cognitive decline by years. Predictive monitoring of neural and autonomic signals reveals early loss of adaptability rather than late-stage impairment.

Vascular aging completes the picture. Blood vessels stiffen, perfusion declines, and tissue oxygenation becomes less reliable. Predictive insight into vascular health predicts not only lifespan, but quality of life.

"Aging accelerates when systems stop speaking to each other."

Reversibility: Where Prediction Becomes Intervention

One of the most powerful insights of longevity science is that early biological aging is often reversible. Predictive science identifies windows where intervention restores coordination rather than merely slowing decline.

Lifestyle interventions guided by predictive insight have measurable impact. Sleep restoration improves metabolic and immune function. Movement restores mitochondrial efficiency and vascular elasticity. Nutritional alignment reduces inflammatory burden. Stress regulation restores autonomic balance. Meaningful engagement preserves neural resilience.

Predictive systems personalize these interventions. Rather than generic advice, individuals receive guidance aligned with their biological trajectory. What slows aging for one person may be ineffective for another. Prediction enables precision longevity.

Emerging therapies amplify this effect. Senolytics target senescent cells. Epigenetic reprogramming shows promise in restoring youthful gene expression patterns. Metabolic modulators enhance cellular efficiency. Predictive science guides their timing, dosage, and candidacy ethically and safely.

Importantly, reversal does not imply erasing age. It implies restoring adaptability. Longevity science values function over appearance, resilience over numbers.

"The goal is not to be younger, but to remain capable."

Longevity, Ethics, and Human Meaning

Longevity science raises profound ethical questions. Extending healthy life reshapes work, family, economics, and identity. Predictive science must guide this transformation responsibly.

Access matters. Longevity interventions must not become privileges of wealth. Ethical longevity prioritizes population health, equity, and dignity.

Psychological impact matters. Prediction of aging trajectories must empower rather than burden. Knowledge of biological age should inspire care, not anxiety.

Meaning matters most. Longevity without purpose is empty. Predictive science must support lives that are not only longer, but richer in connection, creativity, and contribution.

"A longer life is valuable only if it remains a human life."

Toward a Predictive Longevity Future

The future of aging will not be defined by inevitability, but by understanding. Predictive science transforms aging from mystery into measurable process, from passive decline into guided adaptation.

In this future, individuals know their biological trajectory early. Healthcare supports resilience rather than waiting for disease. Societies plan for vitality rather than dependency.

Aging becomes something we participate in consciously, not something that happens to us silently.

Time will still pass. But how we age will no longer be a guess.

"The future of longevity lies not in defeating age, but in understanding it deeply enough to live well within it."

Chapter 38

Predictive Science & The Future of Human Evolution

When Awareness Becomes the Next Step in Evolution

Human evolution has never been a straight line. It has been a dialogue between biology and environment, between challenge and adaptation. For millions of years, evolution unfolded slowly, guided by survival pressures beyond conscious control. Today, something unprecedented is emerging. For the first time, humanity is gaining the ability to **observe its own biological future before it arrives**. Predictive science marks this turning point—not as a force of domination over nature, but as a new form of participation in evolution itself.

This moment should not be met with fear. It should be met with hope. Predictive science does not seek to redesign humanity; it seeks to **understand and protect what makes us human**. It offers the possibility of evolving with awareness rather than suffering through blind trial and error.

"Evolution no longer happens only to us.
It begins to happen with us."

From Survival-Based Evolution to Conscious Adaptation

For most of history, evolution favored traits that maximized survival under harsh conditions. Disease, injury, and scarcity shaped biology ruthlessly.

Today, many of those pressures have shifted. The greatest threats to human health are no longer immediate predators or famine, but chronic disease, environmental stress, psychological overload, and loss of resilience.

Predictive science changes the evolutionary equation. Instead of waiting for breakdown, humanity can identify vulnerability early and respond gently. This is not a rejection of evolution, but its refinement. Evolution becomes less about elimination and more about **preservation of function, diversity, and well-being**.

Biological traits once shaped randomly are now understood systemically. Predictive insight reveals how lifestyle, environment, emotion, and community influence biology across generations. This awareness allows adaptive choices that strengthen resilience without sacrificing individuality.

"The next stage of evolution is not faster bodies,
but wiser adaptation."

Health as an Evolutionary Advantage

In the future shaped by predictive science, health itself becomes an evolutionary advantage—not through competition, but through sustainability. Individuals who understand their biological signals early preserve cognitive clarity, physical capability, and emotional balance across longer lifespans.

This shift has generational impact. Parents who manage health proactively pass on not only genetic material, but epigenetic stability. Children grow up in bodies shaped by balance rather than crisis. Communities become environments that nurture resilience rather than merely manage illness.

Predictive science thus alters evolutionary inheritance. It reduces the burden of preventable disease passed from one generation to the next.

Evolution becomes less about correction through suffering and more about **continuity through care.**

"A healthy future is the most powerful inheritance we can offer."

Technology as a Partner, Not a Replacement

Fears about technology-driven evolution often imagine loss of humanity. Predictive science offers a different vision. Technology does not replace intuition, empathy, or wisdom. It amplifies them.

Predictive systems free humans from constant crisis management, allowing attention to return to creativity, connection, and meaning. When disease is anticipated and softened, life energy shifts from survival toward growth.

Importantly, predictive science values diversity. There is no single optimal human trajectory. Different bodies, minds, and cultures adapt differently. Predictive insight supports personalized paths rather than uniform outcomes.

This partnership between human judgment and technological foresight represents a **co-evolution**, where intelligence evolves not to control life, but to support it.

"Technology evolves best when it remembers who it serves."

Psychological and Social Evolution

Evolution is not only biological. It is psychological and social. Predictive science reduces fear by replacing uncertainty with understanding. When people know that risk can be observed and managed early, anxiety gives way to agency.

Societies evolve as well. Healthcare systems shift from crisis response to long-term stewardship. Education integrates health awareness early. Workplaces support well-being rather than exhaustion. Communities invest in prevention rather than repair.

This evolution fosters compassion. When disease is understood as a process rather than a failure, stigma dissolves. Care becomes collaborative. Responsibility becomes shared.

"Understanding replaces judgment when prediction replaces surprise."

Humanity's Most Hopeful Transition

The future shaped by predictive science is not a world without illness or death. It is a world with **less unnecessary suffering and more informed living**. Aging becomes a guided journey. Disease becomes a signal rather than a catastrophe. Health becomes a dynamic relationship rather than a fragile state.

This transition represents humanity's most hopeful evolutionary step—not toward perfection, but toward awareness. For the first time, the species can sense its own fragility early and respond with intelligence and care.

Evolution no longer waits silently in the background.

It speaks through data, signals, and insight.

Predictive science teaches us to listen.

"The future of humanity will be shaped not by what we can control, but by what we choose to care for."

A Gentle Evolution Forward

Predictive science does not promise a superhuman future. It promises a **more humane one**. A future where children inherit resilience, where adults age with dignity, and where societies grow wiser with time.

Human evolution enters a new chapter—one written not in struggle alone, but in understanding.

And in that understanding, hope finds its strongest foundation.

"The greatest evolution is learning to protect life before it breaks."

Chapter 39

The Next 50 Years: The Age of Intelligent Wellness

When Health Becomes Humanity's Natural State

The next fifty years will mark a quiet revolution—one that may not be remembered for a single invention, discovery, or breakthrough, but for a fundamental shift in how humanity relates to health itself. For centuries, illness has shaped civilization. Wars were paused by epidemics. Economies bent under disease burden. Lives were shortened not by fate, but by late understanding. Predictive science signals the end of this era—not through miracles, but through **awareness, anticipation, and care**.

The Age of Intelligent Wellness does not arrive suddenly. It unfolds gradually, as systems learn to listen earlier and act more gently. It is not a future without medicine, but a future where medicine is guided by foresight rather than urgency. In this world, illness is no longer the primary teacher. Understanding takes its place.

"The greatest healthcare revolution is not curing disease, but preventing suffering."

From Disease-Centered Care to Wellness-Centered Life

For much of history, healthcare revolved around disease. Symptoms defined reality. Diagnosis marked the beginning of care. Treatment followed damage. Predictive science quietly dissolves this sequence. Care begins before symptoms. Health becomes a continuous dialogue rather than an episodic rescue.

In the coming decades, individuals will grow up understanding their bodies as intelligent systems. Subtle signals will be recognized, not ignored. Health education will teach listening rather than fear. Wellness will be dynamic, adaptive, and personal.

This shift changes identity itself. People will no longer define themselves by diagnoses, but by trajectories of resilience. Health will not be measured solely by absence of disease, but by presence of balance, adaptability, and vitality.

"When health becomes visible, illness loses its power."

A Planet That Predicts Before It Suffers

As predictive science scales globally, its impact transcends individual bodies. Entire populations become visible—not as statistics of illness, but as patterns of emerging need. Public health evolves from reaction to anticipation. Outbreaks are sensed before they spread. Chronic disease trends are redirected early. Environmental stressors are identified before they erode biological resilience.

Cities become healthier by design. Workplaces align with human rhythms. Education systems nurture physical and mental resilience alongside intellect. Healthcare becomes woven into daily life rather than confined to institutions.

Even the planet benefits. Reduced disease burden lowers environmental strain from excessive medical intervention. Preventive care aligns naturally with sustainability. A healthier humanity becomes a gentler species.

"An intelligent planet is one that protects life
before life cries for help."

Technology as a Silent Guardian

In the Age of Intelligent Wellness, technology fades into the background. Sensors do not dominate attention. Algorithms do not replace human judgment. Instead, intelligence operates quietly—monitoring, learning, adapting, and intervening only when needed.

Predictive systems act like early immune responses. They detect imbalance, mobilize support, and restore harmony without drama. Health becomes less visible because crisis becomes rare.

Importantly, this intelligence is ethical, transparent, and human-centered. Individuals retain control. Communities retain trust. Technology serves as a guardian, not a master.

"The best technology is the one you forget is protecting you."

Illness as the Exception, Not the Norm

The most radical outcome of predictive science is not longer life alone, but **fewer lives dominated by illness**. Diseases will still exist, but they will be encountered earlier, softened, and often redirected. Aging will continue, but with strength rather than fragility. Mental health will be supported before crisis. Chronic disease will be intercepted before it defines identity.

This does not create a perfect world. It creates a compassionate one—where suffering is reduced not through denial, but through understanding.

Children born into this era inherit not only longer lives, but lighter ones. Lives less interrupted by pain, fear, and uncertainty. Lives free to explore purpose, creativity, and connection.

"A healthy future is one where illness is rare, brief, and never lonely."

Humanity's Quiet Victory

The Age of Intelligent Wellness will not be announced by headlines. It will be noticed slowly—in empty hospital beds, in elders who remain independent, in families spared preventable loss, in communities that thrive quietly.

It will be remembered as the time humanity learned to listen—to biology, to data, to each other. As the moment when intelligence was used not to dominate nature, but to align with it.

This is not the end of medicine.

It is the fulfillment of its deepest promise.

"Medicine succeeds most when it is no longer urgently needed."

Author's Hope

As this book comes to a close, the message is simple and profound: An illness-free planet is not a fantasy.

It is a direction. Predictive science gives humanity the tools to walk that path—with humility, wisdom, and care. The next fifty years belong not to fear of disease, but to confidence in understanding. Not to reaction, but to anticipation. Not to suffering, but to stewardship of life.

The future is not waiting to harm us.

It is waiting to be understood. And in that understanding, humanity finds its greatest healing.

"The healthiest future is the one we choose early—together."

www.ingramcontent.com/pod-product-compliance
Lightning Source LLC
LaVergne TN
LVHW100304210926
848480LV00003B/1022